Bilingual Siblings

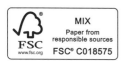

PARENTS' AND TEACHERS' GUIDES
Series Editor: Colin Baker, *Bangor University, UK*

This series provides immediate advice and practical help on topics where parents and teachers frequently seek answers. Each book is written by one or more experts in a style that is highly readable, non-technical and comprehensive. No prior knowledge is assumed: a thorough understanding of a topic is promised after reading the appropriate book.

Full details of all the books in this series and of all our other publications can be found on http://www.multilingual-matters.com, or by writing to Multilingual Matters, St Nicholas House, 31-34 High Street, Bristol BS1 2AW, UK.

PARENTS' AND TEACHERS' GUIDES
Series Editor: Colin Baker, *Bangor University, UK*

Bilingual Siblings
Language Use in Families

Suzanne Barron-Hauwaert

MULTILINGUAL MATTERS
Bristol • Buffalo • Toronto

Library of Congress Cataloging in Publication Data
A catalog record for this book is available from the Library of Congress.
Barron-Hauwaert, Suzanne.
Bilingual Siblings: Language Use in Families/Suzanne Barron-Hauwaert.
Parents' and Teachers' Guides: 12
Includes bibliographical references and index.
1. Bilingualism in children. 2. Brothers and sisters. 3. Families--Language. I. Title.
P115.2.B368 2010
404'.2083–dc22 2010041285

British Library Cataloguing in Publication Data
A catalogue entry for this book is available from the British Library.

ISBN-13: 978-1-84769-327-3 (hbk)
ISBN-13: 978-1-84769-326-6 (pbk)

Multilingual Matters
UK: St Nicholas House, 31–34 High Street, Bristol BS1 2AW, UK.
USA: UTP, 2250 Military Road, Tonawanda, NY 14150, USA.
Canada: UTP, 5201 Dufferin Street, North York, Ontario M3H 5T8, Canada.

The policy of Multilingual Matters/Channel View Publications is to use papers that are natural, renewable and recyclable products, made from wood grown in sustainable forests. In the manufacturing process of our books, and to further support our policy, preference is given to printers that have FSC and PEFC Chain of Custody certification. The FSC and/or PEFC logos will appear on those books where full certification has been granted to the printer concerned.

Typeset by Techset Composition Ltd., Salisbury, UK.
Printed and bound in Great Britain by the MPG Books Group Ltd.

Contents

Contents v

List of Figures

Acknowledgments

I would first like to thank the Multilingual Matters team. I was fortunate to have Colin Baker as my editor and I am grateful for his insights and clarity. The Grover family has played an important role too. Tommi Grover guided the book through to production and Marjukka Grover gave useful feedback on the first draft. For over six years Sami Grover, editor of *The Bilingual Family Newsletter* has commissioned my quarterly column 'Notes from the OPOL Family' where I write about my children and family life in two languages.

I am very grateful to all the multilingual families who replied so promptly to my call for data through *The Bilingual Family Newsletter* and websites around the world. Thanks to the 25 families who took the extra time to give me more information for a case study and reply to all my emails and questions. Their replies and comments formed the basis of the book. Thanks to Sami Grover and Corey Heller from Multilingual Living magazine (www.multilingualliving.com) who helped me reach a wide range of international families for the online survey via their readers.

Thanks to all the parents and teachers who have attended my talks on Family Bilingualism or have joined the Bilingual Support Groups I ran in Kuala Lumpur and France over the last seven years. Your stories and experiences were important and have percolated through into this book. Thanks to all my wonderful friends around the world; Kuala Lumpur's multilingual cooking group, French *mamans* in Chicago and my English friends here in France. Your chats over coffee inspired me and I hope some of my advice helped your families. Thanks to Sharon and June for their proof-reading of the first draft.

Closer to home I would like to say *merci* to Jacques, my French husband, for his critical support and computer help. Last, but not least, my three amazing children,

Marc, 13, Nina, 11 and Gabriel, 7, who have provided me with working models of various stages of bilingualism over time. I would like to say thank you to all their hard-working teachers and assistants over the last 10 years, who have dealt with various stages of language refusal, mixed language and speech problems.

As this book goes to print we are living in rural France and our three children are all attending French schools here. My children continue to surprise me with their ability to use two languages on a daily basis and feel at home in many cultures. It is with great pride that I see them making friends in both languages, maintaining links with their grandparents and cousins in two languages and feeling at home in two very different countries. Bravo!

http://opol-family.blogspot.com

Introduction

This book is all about bilingual and multilingual families; the parents, their children and their choice of languages. The languages a child hears and speaks can be passed on by a parent, or linked to a place or a country. The emergence of two or more languages is a wonderful thing to witness in a child's world and the languages can be mixed together or used in separate situations or locations. As children grow up bilingually, parents can observe how their children fluidly switch from language to language to communicate with both sides of the family or within the community where they live. How do parents prepare for the arrival of a child in a bilingual family or community? Academic studies and books for parents are available to support parents and to guide them through the child's first words and dual language use. However, studies rarely go beyond the first child starting school and often by this time a second or third child has joined the family the parents have usually established the way they communicate with their children, and a clear family language pattern exists. How do siblings fit into this family language pattern? Do all the siblings follow the same language model or do they adapt language use to suit their own needs? Will one or more child refuse to speak one language? Will two children living in the same home, with the same parents and language input, grow up with identical or have different ways of communicating linguistically? Sibling language use remains a mystery.

We know very little about the dynamics of bilingual children's speech and how they communicate away from the influence of parents. In this book you will see how within a bilingual or multilingual family the siblings generally all speak the same languages, but not always. One child might prefer to use more or less of the mother's or father's language. One or more children might be more comfortable speaking the language of the school, or the community where they live. A bilingual family's biggest challenge is to provide enough exposure to each language, to ensure each child not only hears both languages but has a chance to speak and practice too. This book explains how siblings communicate in two or more languages, within the bilingual and multilingual family setting.

TWO OR MORE CHILDREN

Siblings are the brothers and sisters in a family. It is estimated that 80% of children in the United States or Europe have a sibling. Around 10% of families have five or more children and about 1% of all births are twins. According to a study released in 2006, the average American family has 2.1 children. In 2008, statistics showed that European women have an average of 1.5 children, with a birth rate that has been falling for 30 years (except in France and Spain). In general terms, Canada, Western Europe, Australia, the Baltic States and China have declining birth rates of less than two children per family. Growing populations of families with three children are found in North and South Africa, along with some southeastern states in America. Central Africa and some parts of South-East Asia have rapidly growing birth rates. Some brothers and sisters have similar personalities and features, while others may be very different physically or in character. They may have the same parents, or they may be part of a family which encompasses half-brothers or sisters or step-siblings from widowed or divorced parents. There are also families who have adopted or fostered children.

To investigate how children interact with each other we have to look at the work of child psychologists. This field of research closely observes children's behavior and their developing relationships with the people around them. Over the last century, psychologists have investigated the influence of working parents, stay-at-home mothers, absent fathers, child-minders and early schooling, often with contradictory findings. Their results and conclusions can be passed on to parents via doctors and health workers, often in the form of advice or parenting guides or through parenting magazines or television programs. Recommendations to parents such as being strict and disciplined, or allowing the child to choose when they sleep or what they eat can have serious ramifications on sensitive young children. Recent research into children has focused on the genetic makeup of a child and how genes might affect the personality of the child, for example, whether a child is 'programmed' to be active or passive. There are also developmental psychologists who look at the effect of the environment, such as the child's home, school or their parent's education and background. The debate over how the mix of a child's inherited character traits, environmental influences and family makeup forms a child's character, is ongoing. One thing that the psychologists do agree on is that parenting is a gamble, and what works well with one child may not suit another.

In general, siblings are rather under-researched, compared to the vast amount of work done on the mother–child relationship and the effect of the peer group on children. Interestingly, some children spend more time with their siblings than with their parents, and a sibling can play the role of surrogate parent, teacher, playmate or friend. However, a sibling usually has less dominance than a parent because he or she is closer to the other children in terms of behavior. Siblings can be close and care deeply about each other, but there can be intense rivalry, competition and jealousy over people, property or rights, which creates tension at home. Nevertheless, we must remember that siblings are in a 'non-voluntary' relationship, and usually have no choice about their parent's decision to have other children. Siblings are unable to escape each other at home, and may be obliged to share a room, toys or space. To get the best out of the forced sibling relationship, children must learn how to live and learn together. Psychologists agree that older siblings typically play the role of a teacher and are a strong role model for a younger sibling. The younger siblings often take the role of pupil and look for help or assistance (with games, writing or reading) from older family members. A younger sibling likes to imitate and interact with their older brother or sister, but can be overly dependent on their brother or sister, to the exclusion of other children. Siblings can form a very strong emotional attachment with their baby brother or sister, and protect them from danger or harm. Children learn, through their siblings, how to negotiate and resolve problems and to see things from another person's perspective. However, they often turn out with very different characters and personalities. Long-term studies completed by researchers working closely with families conclude that even siblings living together and sharing the same experiences can turn out as different as two children raised in two different environments.

Articles cited

USA birth statistics:

On WWW at http://www.census.gov/population/www/cen2000/briefs.html. Accessed 10.3.10.

On WWW at www.usatoday.com/news/nation/2007-12-19-fertility_N.htm

'Fertility rate in USA on upswing' by Haya El Nasser and Paul Overberg. Accessed 10.3.10.

European birth statistics:

On WWW at http://europa.eu/rapid/pressReleasesAction.do?reference= MEMO/05/96&format=HTML&aged=0&language=EN&guiLanguage=en. Accessed 25.4.08.

'Europe's changing population structure and its impact on relations between the generations' (2005).

World family birth statistics:

On WWW at http://www.pregnantpause.org/numbers/fertility.htm. Accessed 10.3.10.

'Fertility Rates (Children per Family) World Statistics' (2001).

SIBLINGS IN BILINGUAL OR MULTILINGUAL FAMILIES

What is a bilingual or multilingual family? It is a family where two or more languages are used regularly. Within the bilingual family there are many different variations – two parents with different languages, a family living in a second-language country, a parent using a second language with their children or a family living in a community or a country which has two languages. When a second child joins a bilingual family, parents are delighted to watch the now fluently bilingual first child teach the new baby words or songs that they learnt just a few years ago. In many families the second or subsequent children become as linguistically competent as their big brothers and sisters and benefit greatly from the child-friendly conversation and role-modeling the sibling gives. But what happens if the second child does not turn out to be as fluent in both languages as the first one? What happens when one child refuses to speak one language, while the other one speaks it fluently? What if one has a perfect accent while the other sounds like a tourist in his own country? How do we react when we see one child mixing the languages and the other keeping the languages separate? These are questions asked by parents around the world.

Take the five following real-life examples.

Lise is the fourth child of French-English parents who lived in England. In England in the 1970s, the French mother wanted to fit in with her new country and life, and felt uncomfortable speaking French in public. In private, the French mother chatted to her first-born child and passed on her love of French nursery rhymes. But by the time Lise arrived, the house was full of English-speaking siblings, local friends visiting to play and a mother who spoke mostly English at home too. Lise understands French but does not speak it and now regrets never getting the same input her older sisters and brothers had. Now a mother of four children herself, Lise is hoping they will have the chance to speak more French than she did, and they regularly go to France on holiday or to visit French family.

Corinne is a bilingual French mother married to a Scotsman. Their first son, Brice, went to a local school in Scotland. Although she had always spoken to him in French, Corinne found that eight-year-old Brice would not speak French, although he understood it. When the family moved to Malaysia in 2003, they chose an English-language school for Brice and decided to put their four-year-old daughter, Chloe, in a French-language preschool. Corinne wanted at least one of her children to speak French. Chloe loved the French school and made several French friends, while still maintaining her English through friends from the condo where she lived. However, after two years of juggling two very different schools, Corinne decided to transfer Chloe to the British primary school. Meanwhile, Brice had become more positive toward French. When the family bought a house near their family in France for summer holidays, Brice found a reason to practice his emerging French. Now both children have made friends in the village and chat together in French.

Mazdida is a Malaysian married to a Frenchman with three children, Adam, Pierre and Camilla. Mazdida spoke in the local Bahasa Malaya dialect of Malaysia; her husband spoke French, while English was the main language of communication between the couple. The first son, Adam, flourished, and after English preschool was transferred to a French primary school where he did very well. When they put their second son, Pierre, in the French school three years later it was a different story. Pierre refused to speak French to the French-speaking class teacher. At a parent–teacher meeting, the father wondered why his son could not understand French at school. When the teacher asked them how much French Pierre spoke at home, the parents realized that they had all started speaking English at home, without noticing. With time alone speaking just French with his Papa, and a month long trip to France, Pierre improved. Pierre is now able to participate in classes normally.

Elisabeth is a French national living in New York with three children, Thomas, Heloise and Theodore. Her French husband loves America and wants the kids to grow up bilingual. When they arrived in New York in 2004, four-year-old Thomas had already established his French and quickly picked up English in the local kindergarten. However, his two-year-old sister, Heloise, refused to talk at all and blocked out both languages. When Heloise began to talk it was in English, the language of the crèche where she spent most days, although she understood French. The father spoke mostly English with the children too, proud that he was bringing up his children bilingually. In 2006 Thomas started attending a bilingual French/English primary school and the linguistic balance changed at home, as Thomas brought French homework and French-speaking friends to play. Heloise now felt comfortable trying out some French words with her brother. For the first time, the siblings spoke French together at home.

Raul, an American lawyer in Chicago, of Mexican descent, is proud of his family heritage. Like many Mexican-American families, he notes that the use of Spanish is decreasing, to the shame of his family. Chicago has a high Mexican origin population, yet 96% of Chicanos living there prefer to speak English. Raul says that his older brother only learnt Spanish curse words, while he learnt just enough to pass at school, and his younger brother did not learn Spanish at all. Even though their mother pushed them to watch bilingual news stations, the three teenage boys were not motivated to actually speak Spanish and read or write in the language. Now, as an adult, he is making an effort to learn his grandparent's language and is taking courses and looking for ways to practice Spanish in the community.

The siblings in Lise, Corinne, Mazdida, Elisabeth and Raul's families show the different experiences and reactions can have to their linguistic heritage. Each child arrives in a family with established language patterns and expectations. Over time, the parents evolve and adapt their original language choices to fit in with changing circumstances. How do we reconcile our evolving parenting with establishing bilingualism in the family? Do our family strategies change as the family grows? Do we stop being strict with language use and accept grammatical errors that we never let the first one make? How does the language of the older child affect the younger one? Does the older sibling take the role of parent-teacher for one or more languages? Will an older sibling make fun of a younger child's mistakes? As the children grow up they make linguistic decisions for themselves that leave the parents feeling powerless and unable to intervene or choose the language the siblings choose to speak in. These issues will be considered throughout the book.

WHO THIS BOOK IS FOR

The book is aimed primarily at parents with two or more children living in a bilingual environment. Parents may already be bringing up their children bilingually, or wondering how they can help improve, encourage or maintain bilingual language use in their home. The book is also useful for people working directly with bilingual and multilingual children; teachers, classroom assistants, counselors and speech therapists. This book brings together the experiences of over a hundred real bilingual families taken from an online internet survey, detailed case studies from around the globe and current research on multilingualism. From informal website discussion groups to organized seminars and workshops, parents wonder how they can facilitate the best language environment within their particular family. The majority of the important academic research on bilingualism over the last century was carried on first-borns or only children. Although this research is still valid we need to include families with two, three or more children. We also need to consider parents who may or may not be living together, step-parents and step-siblings, and the important people in the child's world, the teachers, daycare workers, tutors, nannies and babysitters. All of these people might affect the child's decision to use or refuse to use a language.

As an independent researcher, I focus on the bilingual family as a whole. As a parent of three children, I regularly hear bilingual and multilingual concerns, and the uncertainty of parenting in two languages. Parents can be geographically divided from whole branches of their families and lack people to talk to in their first language. Others can struggle to keep their children academically on track in one language while supporting another language at home or through the community. Some parents are communicating with their children in their second language. There are parents who wonder why their second or third child uses their languages in a different way and what they can do to help all their children become bilingual. The influence of siblings on each other has hardly been studied at all and it is time to hear about the language development of all children and the sibling dynamics that are created within the family.

The groundwork for our knowledge on how bilingual children develop has been done over the last hundred years, by respected academic linguists such as Werner

Leopold, Jules Ronjat, George Saunders, Alvino Fantini, Traute Taeschner and Stephen Caldas. The majority of these researchers studied their own children at home, giving a detailed description of home life with two languages. There are also important studies carried out by independent researchers, comparing children or looking for wider trends within bilingual families. In Chapter 1, you can read more about their case studies, and how they have helped us understand more about how bilingualism works within the family. Throughout the book I will refer to the academic studies and how they link to family bilingualism.

The book begins with a selection of questions on siblings and multilingualism. Chapter 1 is all about what we know about bilingual families, with a brief review of important and relevant academic studies and books on bilingual parenting. Chapter 2 looks at the growing family and the strategies they can employ to suit their language needs. In Chapters 3 through 7, we discuss factors which may have an influence on siblings and their consequent language use: sibling relationships, age gaps, family size, gender, birth order and individual personality differences. These six factors are linked to bilingualism and language use, with examples from case studies and families who participated in a survey. Chapter 8 discusses families with specific issues, such as twins, step-children or adopted siblings. Chapter 9 has an overview of the main five themes.

THREE VERY DIFFERENT SIBLINGS

My children are the inspiration for my research into bilingualism and multilingualism. I am English and my husband, Jacques, is French. Together we generally speak English. As a teacher of English as a Second Language before starting a family, I knew how children could progress from beginners to fluent speakers in a short time. I was sure that for our children bilingualism would be a given certainty. I had many questions about bilingualism, which led to a Masters course in Education, and a dissertation on trilingual families two years later. In 2001, I began to research language strategies, based on my personal experiences and those of families around the world following one parent-one language (OPOL) or other family strategies. The result was the book *Language Strategies for Bilingual Families – The One Parent One Language Approach* (2004). My research showed that bringing up children bilingually is like any aspect of parenting, and there is no guarantee a child will become bilingual even with the best of intentions and materials.

Our first son was born in 1997. We had begun like many families with a clear decision to follow the OPOL strategy, which was frequently recommended in parenting books. Consequently, I only spoke English to Marc and Jacques spoke French. However, I found OPOL did not always fit our needs, especially when we were with friends or family who found it strange that we only spoke one language to our child. At two years and four months, Marc was just beginning to string two words together when his sister, Nina, was born in 1999 in Zurich, Switzerland. He was looked after by a Swiss-German child-minder three mornings a week and a French-speaking babysitter some afternoons. Marc was a quiet child and managed to communicate well with gestures, smiles and a limited amount of words. Like many older siblings, his speech regressed with the arrival of the new baby in our home and because we had less time to talk or read to him directly.

We moved to France when Marc was three years and three months old, and when he started going to a French preschool (*école maternelle*) he began to talk. Marc's English was quite good for his age, and he had just enough French to communicate with his cousins and at school. Around the same time, one-year-old Nina began to talk, with a mix of French and English that would be her trademark, and for the first time the two siblings began to play together and chat, both in English and French. A move to England a year later meant formal English schooling for Marc and Nina. French faded away within a few months, while Marc and Nina's level of English skyrocketed as they made local friends and settled into life in England. Nina became a chatty and articulate little girl at preschool. But her French remained 'baby talk' and she preferred to speak English rather than not be able to communicate in French fluently. Even with frequent trips to France and French visitors, Nina made virtually no progress from the words she had learnt as a toddler. We were concerned when three-year-old Nina began answering her French father and her French grandparents in English. Marc had never done that before, and to us it seemed disappointing that she would reply in the 'wrong' language after all our efforts to cultivate bilingualism through the OPOL approach.

In reality, the balance had changed within the family and we had not responded to it. French was no longer the majority language of communication; the only people who used French were Marc and his Papa. Marc and Nina spoke mainly in English at home, because the children they played with after school only spoke English. Nina was bright enough to see that Papa obviously understood English too and there was no need for her to speak French with him. We had reached an important stage in our bilingual family. We had the choice of changing to a *minority-language-at-home* strategy (where Jacques, Marc and I would only speak French at home). In theory, this could push Nina to speak French, but would demand me speaking my rather weak second language with my husband and son. Or we had the choice of returning to live in France, with French schools and support from the family.

Work intervened in the end when Jacques was posted to Kuala Lumpur, Malaysia at the end of 2002. In Malaysia, English is widely spoken and taught at local schools. However, for religious and cultural reasons, most expatriates choose an international school for their children. Seeing that French was on the decline and we would be living far away from the French family we decided to enroll Marc and Nina in the *Lycée Français*, a private French-language school in Kuala Lumpur. Marc settled in quickly, his French language was still operational and he only had a few problems with pronunciation of unfamiliar sounds when he was reading. On the other hand, four-year-old Nina was furious to be dropped into the French system and reacted strongly to having to speak French all day. Marc was there to help her at school in the first trimester and he would translate words and phrases for her. Returning to school after the long summer holidays Nina spontaneously switched to French. Within a few weeks she found herself two or three French friends and began to play with Marc in French. Then to our amazement, she started speaking English with a French accent, presumably to fit in with her French friends. This was something Marc had never done, and we always took pride in his clear British accent. Nothing could persuade Nina otherwise and she continued to speak in her own way. But at least both children were speaking both languages and we were happy with our choice of school.

In 2003, Gabriel joined the family. The four-year age difference between Nina, and six years between Marc, meant he was more alone with me, since the others were at school five days a week. By the time he started speaking, we were finally in a relatively balanced French-English household, where his two siblings had established their bilingualism. The family strategy was moving from the stricter 'OPOL' to a more 'mixed' strategy. Jacques and I had become more relaxed about which language each person spoke, we allowed Marc and Nina to mix or choose either language, confident that they would use the right language when they had to (which they usually did). With two children in the French school, I began speaking more French with teachers and the other parents, and my level of French dramatically improved. On holiday in France, I now spoke French with the children in front of my French family and friends and even to Jacques. We thought that bilingualism was a given. Two out of our three children had become bilingual, even with a few teething problems. We had managed to convince the in-laws, the teachers and the doctors that we were on the right track. So we rested on our laurels and watched Marc and Nina teach Gabriel.

Gabriel was a quick learner and some of his first words were naughty words, taught by his big brother and sister. He started going to an English language pre-school three days a week at age two in Kuala Lumpur. He had two or three French-speaking friends, often brothers or sisters of his siblings' friends. We soon noticed that Gabriel forced them all to speak English, even if it was just 'yes' or 'no'. Gabriel also spoke only English with Jacques, but in an even more pronounced way than Nina, he would not even let Jacques speak French back to him. Jacques succumbed and replied in English, breaking the golden rule of OPOL that we had so carefully followed for seven years. A year living in America after we left Malaysia did not help either. Gabriel was too young to attend the bilingual French-English school his siblings went too and was even more immersed in English. At age three his spoken French was limited and something had to be done.

In 2007 we came back to live in France and this time Gabriel had a linguistic shock. Like Nina, he had to readjust and learn to use his father's language at school and with the family. But curiously he spoke French with an English accent, the reverse of Nina's French-accented English. As I write this Marc is a teenager, and in *collège*, or secondary school, and he still clearly separates the two languages and cultures and sees himself as having two identities. He rarely mixes and has very good accents in both languages. Marc likes to correct his sibling's language use. Nina continues to mix the two languages in her own unique way, dropping in French words in practically every English sentence, and has a cultural leaning toward France more than England. Nina's French-accented English can be a barrier with her English friends but she prefers it like that. Marc and Nina talk together in a mix of English and French, depending on the subject. They both read in either language. Meanwhile Gabriel, who attends primary school and is learning his first letters and words, remains the baby of the family. He clearly understands French very well, and is very communicative, but he continues to have a strange accent and now is seeing a speech therapist to correct his articulation.

Are our family's language patterns affected by birth-order, gender, personality or sibling rivalry? Why does Marc make the effort to speak correctly? Is Nina's mixing just a way to be different from her older brother or linked to her personality? Should we have spent more time helping Gabriel with his language development? These are questions I have not yet found the answers to. How could three children with the same parental languages be so different? I have not scientifically tested or made detailed or comparative studies on my children, like some of the well-known parent-linguists such as Werner Leopold, Traute Taeschner, Antonio Fantini, George Saunders and Steven Caldas (see Chapter 1 for more on these studies). I greatly admire their in-depth longitudinal studies, which shed light on the specific linguistic side of family interactions and they inform this book. Nevertheless, since my children could speak I have made brief notes regarding their first words and phrases and their reaction to starting school or interaction with family and friends. I have written about my children's linguistic milestones, cultural misunderstandings, sibling interactions and their social adaptations to English and French (and other languages that we have come into contact with over the last decade). These observations are published in my quarterly column 'Notes from the OPOL Family' in *The Bilingual Family Newsletter*[1] and my blog: 'Notes from the OPOL Family'.[2] The column and blog chronicle the linguistic ups and downs of our family. Although I do not offer a scientific linguistic or psychological analysis, my observations are based on 12 years of closely watching sibling interaction within my family and observing the siblings of numerous bilingual and multilingual families I know around the world.

(1) *The Bilingual Family Newsletter* – a quarterly magazine for bilingual families published by Multilingual Matters. (Ended December 2010 but archive available at www.bilingualfamilynewsletter.com/archives.php)
(2) Blog: 'Notes from the OPOL Family' http://opol-family.blogspot.com

QUESTIONS ON FAMILY LANGUAGE USE

Here are a selection of questions asked by parents on the subject of family bilingualism and siblings, with links to the appropriate chapters for more information. These questions have been taken from parenting chat forums, bilingual websites and from my personal experience discussing bilingualism with families from around the world. They are anonymous questions, and any advice is given in general terms and does not necessarily apply to all families.

Should we adapt our family strategies as the family grows?

A strategy chosen when we have a baby or very young child may not be applicable with a school age or adolescent child. Rather strict and rigid strategies like OPOL or *minority-language-at-home* work well with young children, but might backfire when older children understand that their parents understand each other's language. Older children might prefer to speak the language of the school or community at home. External factors like relocating to a new country or school with a different language can affect the balance of each language in the home. Parents do need to adapt as their family grows and discuss with their children the cultural value and importance of maintaining a parental or heritage language.

Note: See Chapter 2 for more on family strategies.

Our children do not want us to speak the minority language with them, what should we do?

Children's needs and perception of a language can change over time. They may feel uncomfortable or embarrassed in front of their school or friends when a parent speaks a minority language and prefer to be 'monolingual'. Parents can discuss the importance of bilingualism with their children, depending on their age, in terms of their heritage, family, educational or economic reasons. If speaking a language to please a parent is not enough, the parents may need other solutions outside the home, such as language classes, camps and activities, where links with other children can give a reason for children speaking that language. Children's friendships and social lives can often support a language as strongly as a parent can.

Note: See Chapters 2 and 3 for more on maintaining a minority language.

What language will our children speak together?

In the early years, a parental language is the strongest influence: but when children start school or increase their social links with the community they tend to choose the language of the country or the school so their preferred language can change as they grow. Many siblings enjoy mixing together; because they understand both languages this is a linguistic game they can play. Siblings may revert to their minority language in public, so as to have a private conversation. Parents cannot really control their children's language choice, it is up to them and we should respect their choice. The choice or 'preference' is a practical one for the siblings as a group; all siblings need to be able to speak that language, and it makes sense if they can also speak that language with their friends too. Parents concerned about sibling language preferences may need to rethink the school or country language, and the future effect on the children.

Note: See Chapter 3 for more on sibling language choices.

How do we react when we see one of our children mixing up the languages?

Mixing at an early age is a normal part of a child's bilingual development. Older children choose to mix as a sophisticated feature often heard between bilinguals. Some children will separate each language clearly, while others will add in a phrase or word from the other language. There can be a difference between the way parents accept or allow mixing. Parents should not worry as long as the child uses the right language with the right person.

Note: See Chapter 3 for more on mixing.

How does the number of children affect bilingualism in the family?

One child will hear more adult conversation, possibly leading to a broader vocabulary and a more sophisticated grammar. He or she will be able to ask more questions and have more one-to-one time with the parents. Two or more siblings may have less direct adult–child talk, but can benefit from child-to-child-talk. Watching and listening in to siblings using two languages can help a younger sibling 'learn the ropes'. They will also learn how to interrupt, argue and probably learn a few slang or swearwords in each language as well.

Note: See Chapter 4 for more on family size.

Can an older sibling help teach a language to a younger child?

Big sisters seem to love 'teaching' their younger siblings and this natural interest can be beneficial in supporting a weaker or minority language. Children may share their love of songs, movies and books with a new baby. However, we should not leave the teaching to siblings, because children need a whole range of language models. Parents should be careful of big sisters not taking their role too far, and talking for or translating for a younger sibling.

Note: See Chapter 4 for more on inter-sibling teaching.

Will the age gap of our children matter in language use?

Close-in-age siblings tend to share more things and have a similar lifestyle and attend school together. Language has an important role in their games and everyday communication. Children with a gap of six or more years might have more separate lives, but the older one is more likely to teach a younger child.

Note: See Chapter 4 for more on age.

Do girls speak earlier than boys?

Girls generally speak a little earlier than boys and are often more interested in small social groups, where talking and communicating are important skills for making friends. Boys may be more interested in physical and active skills at an early age. By the time boys and girls reach the end of primary school their linguistic skills are usually at the same level.

Note: See Chapter 5 for more on gender.

Does being a boy or a girl make a difference in the way our children communicate in bilingual terms?

Girls may be judged as becoming bilingual earlier. Conversely, boys can be seen as lacking bilingual speech in the preschool years. The age when children start using two languages is not so important in the long run; the main issue is how to keep children speaking two languages. Parents with girls should not be over confident that their daughters will stay bilingual and parents with boys should not give up if their son is not speaking two languages at an early age. In some languages, such as Hebrew, there is gender-specific language use. A child might not have enough exposure to models of female or male language use and can sound wrong. Parents need to give a wide variety of language examples to their children.

Note: See Chapter 5 for more on gender.

Does birth order affect bilingualism in the family?

Psychologists are wary of giving much credence to birth order. What they do agree on is that first-borns tend to dominate their siblings, while middle ones look for a different way to please their parents and last-born children may try to keep the role of 'baby' as long as they can and use their status to get attention. Sibling dominance appears to be particularly strong within the home. An older first-born child may have a wider vocabulary and may try harder to be correct when they speak or write. This does not mean that younger siblings cannot achieve the same proficiency. Younger siblings may benefit from having a model of a child speaking each language. Young siblings can feel less pressure to be correct and have a more creative approach to language.

Note: See Chapter 6 for more on birth order.

What should we do if our children tease or laugh at other's linguistic mistakes?

Siblings are known to correct, laugh at the other's linguistic mistakes or put down a sister or brother who is trying to say something. In bilingual terms, a sibling can feel undermined when using a language they are not fluent or confident in. It can also lead to a sibling using less of one language or stopping speaking it if they feel upset.

Note: See Chapter 6 for more on language friction.

What do we do when one child refuses to speak one language, while the other one speaks it perfectly?

This problem can be due to siblings unconsciously competing, especially when they are the same gender or close in age. If one child cannot be as good as his older sibling, he may decide to do the opposite. Parents need to remember that not all siblings have the same linguistic abilities, like musical and artistic talents. Sometimes a child may feel more culturally attached to one language or country and over time the other language can become passive or under-used. A child can also feel he can never catch up in one language, and decide to 'drop' one language. Parents need to find out why the child will not speak the language and try to support and encourage the child.

Note: See Chapter 7 for more on individual differences.

How can two children living in the same home and having the same language input end up so different linguistically?

Siblings sharing a home and having the same parental language input are affected by the way they learn, the opportunities they are given to practice language and the feedback they receive when they speak each language. Even twins with the same genes and environment can turn out differently. A second child arrives in a family with an established strategy, but each child approaches a language from a different perspective. As parents, we may think we provide exactly the same language environment, but in reality, each child brings a new dimension to the family and increases or decreases overall language use in one or more languages.

Note: See Chapter 7 for more on individual differences.

Chapter 1
What Do We Know about Bilingual Families?

In this chapter we briefly examine the important academic work that has been published on bilingual and multilingual families over the last hundred years. There are some fascinating studies on the interaction of children being brought up with two languages. The majority of academic studies describe the language development of a first-born or only child. Why has research on bilingualism only focused on one child? Has any research been done on bilingual and multilingual siblings? A small number of studies followed bilingual sibling language patterns and were typically conducted by bilingual linguists or researchers describing their own children. Werner Leopold, Alvino Fantini, George Saunders, Traute Taeschner, Charlotte Hoffmann, Harriet Jisa, Stephen Caldas and Madalena Cruz-Ferreira dedicated their time to transcribing the language use of their children.

Complementing the diary studies were several respected academic researchers working from different perspectives. From a sociolinguistic point of view, Christine Helot, Masayo Yamamoto and Susanne Döpke observed bilingual families in Ireland, Japan and Australia. Education specialists, Eve Gregory and Victoria Obied, tracked the literacy patterns and language use of bilingual siblings in London and Portugal. Books aimed at parents and educators, which discussed sibling relationships, were authored by Colin Baker, Una Cunningham-Andersson, Tracey Tokuhama-Espinosa, Edith Harding and Philip Riley, Kendall King and Alison Mackay and Barbara Zuer-Pearson.

THE LACK OF SIBLING SETS IN ACADEMIC RESEARCH

When I began reading studies of bilingual children, one of the first things I noticed was that they usually deal with only one child. Typically, biographical or case studies document the speech patterns of a first-born or only child, usually under the age of five. Annick de Houwer, Margaret Deucher, Elizabeth Lanza and Susanne Döpke are highly respected researchers who focused on one child in a home environment and revealed their early bilingual development. Researchers have their reasons for only focusing on one child. In the early days, they had to write each word phonetically, making the process very lengthy. Transcribing a child's actual words into text is still a long process, even though we now have the possibility to record or video a child, which gives us the chance to rewind and check exactly what they said. If you try to write down just 10 minutes of a young child's conversation you will soon find that you are scribbling fast, making abbreviations and often missing parts of a sentence. When recording a child at home a researcher also needs to know who the child is talking to, what the child is talking about, and explain any specific references to family or friends. So we can understand why the researchers preferred that another sibling was not around to interrupt their dialogue, change the language or the subject of the conversation. It also explains why much of the research is on young preschool children, who are usually two or three years old, and have a limited vocabulary or lower word counts. It is also much harder to record the conversations of children talking to other children, with their fast-paced chat, playground slang, jokes and expressions that only they understand. Siblings can be even more idiosyncratic, with made-up words, songs, stories, or even occasionally with twins, made-up languages that they use together. To untangle such fast communication for analysis is a challenge.

University-based large-scale linguistic and psychological tests were also conducted from the 1960s onwards with bilingual children. The research was conducted in scientific laboratories with carefully selected children, observing a child in isolation from their siblings. Researchers tested a child's knowledge of grammar and vocabulary in one or both languages and their ability to switch from language to language. The tests were controlled with a group of children of the same age or similar language ability who were specifically chosen for comparison. Each child received the same test and their results were compared and analyzed for common errors or reactions. Including a sibling in tests would skew the results, simply because they are younger or older (unless it was an identical twin). A sibling might not have the same intellectual abilities, for example, four-year-olds make mistakes with verb endings or irregular verbs saying 'I goed to school' instead of 'I went to school' and it would not be fair to compare a seven-year-old with a five-year-old sibling. Thus, researchers tend to use a homogenous selection of children for study in a laboratory. The chances of finding 20 children with siblings of the same age, gender and educational level would be low. Therefore, what we know about siblings generally comes from parent-linguist's reports or from selected case studies on two or three children in the same family.

PARENT RESEARCHERS AND DIARY DATA

There are several detailed diaries or journals of individual children written by parents who are academic researchers in the field of linguistics. One of the first biographical works was compiled by linguist Jules Ronjat (1913) on his bilingual son Louis and the linguist Werner Leopold began a four-volume series of books on his first-born daughter, Hildegard in the 1940s. These case studies often span 10 or more years, from first words up to primary education, or in some cases through the teenage years. Werner Leopold, Alvino Fantini, George Saunders, Traute Taeschner, Charlotte Hoffmann, Harriet Jisa, Madalena Cruz-Ferreira and Stephen Caldas have all recorded authentic child speech in their own homes, with two or more children. Their observations give us an insight into bilingual child development. In this chapter, I will give you a brief summary of these eight real-life bilingual family stories, which are accessible to read via a good university linguistics library.

The Leopold family: Hildegard and her papa

One of the earliest records of child speech was by the famous linguist Werner Leopold (*Speech Development of a Bilingual Child: A Linguist's Record*, 1939–1949). While working at Northwestern University in America he spent almost 20 years tracing the language development of his English/German bilingual daughter's speech patterns. Born in 1930, Hildegard grew up in America with second-generation German heritage parents. The Leopold family followed the OPOL strategy, which was first described in 1902 by the French linguist Jules Grammont. Inspired by Grammont, Werner decided to try the strategy, with himself as the main source of German in the family. Werner described in great detail the utterances and mixes of the two languages that Hildegard made from age two months to around age seven, with follow-up diary excerpts into her teenage years. In bilingual terms, Hildegard was a great success and her speech mirrored the developmental milestones of a monolingual child. Leopold had another daughter

---

Werner F. Leopold

Speech Development of a Bilingual Child:
A Linguists Record
1939–1949

Biographical data on his daughter
  Hildegard, with some notes on
  sibling, Karla, 6 yrs younger
From birth – 7 yrs, and later recordings
  up to 15 yrs

Mother – English
Father – German/English

Family living in America
Strategy: OPOL

too, Karla, who was six years younger than Hildegard. Karla was not so keen to speak German as her sister. When Karla was five Werner noted,

> Karla's German is extremely limited. She scatters some German words over her English sentences when she speaks to me, as a sort of concession to my way of speaking. (Werner, 1949b: 159)

Karla appeared to be less keen to speak German to her father than her sister and we do not know if Karla mixed languages because she lacked German vocabulary, or to upset her father. Perhaps Karla's refusal to speak fully in German with her father was a reaction to her older sister's linguistic prowess, since Werner disapproved of mixing. On the other hand Karla mixed languages with her bilingual sister Hildegard and found it natural. In the end, the two girls evened out, with Karla speaking German perfectly when she visited family in Germany, and Hildegard leaning more toward English as her dominant language.

The Fantini family and their Latino environment

Like Werner Leopold, Alvino Fantini (*Language Acquisition of a Bilingual Child*, 1985) was a linguist who recorded the language development of his son, Mario, from his first words to around age ten. His book was originally his PhD dissertation at the University of Texas. An American with Italian heritage, Alvino spoke Italian and Spanish at home, alongside several other languages. His wife was from South America and was fluent in English, Spanish, Italian and Portuguese. The family lived in America and Alvino chose to speak one of his wife's languages, Spanish, to his children to maintain her Latino heritage. The parents wanted Mario to grow up speaking Spanish fluently and chose the *minority-language at home* strategy, to help him acquire Spanish before starting at a local English-language school in America. The parents benefited from being able to spend long periods of time with the maternal Spanish-speaking family, and they employed several Spanish speaking nannies who lived with them.

> **Alvino E. Fantini**
>
> *Language Acquisition of a Bilingual Child. A Sociolinguistic Perspective*
> 1985
>
> Biographical data on son, Mario and details on younger sister, Carla
> From age birth to age 10
>
> Mother – Portuguese/Spanish/Italian/English
> Father – English (of Italian descent)
> Family living in America
>
> Strategy: Minority Language at Home (Spanish)

Alvino remarked that, 'The child {Mario} received considerable attention, not only because he was the first and only child for a time, but also because he had a nursemaid {Spanish-speaking} who was entirely dedicated to him'. This is typical in

Bolivian families and is an important factor, because Mario often spent '... more contact hours on a daily basis with the nursemaid than he did with his parents'. Like Hildegard, Mario was a linguist prodigy and quickly picked up the two languages with apparent ease. Alvino credits the success to regular trips to visit his wife's family in Bolivia and Mexico, and Mario's own cultural interest in languages and communication.

Mario's sister, Carla, was born when he was four years and four months, just a few months after Mario had declared '*Yo hablo dos*' (I have two languages), which had delighted his parents. Mario is described as being protective and caring toward her. Alvino observed that Mario,

> ... spoke to his sister in his usual manner, without a distinct style shift, except when displaying affection in which case he invoked a style of Spanish he had heard adults use when speaking to children. (Fantini, 1985: 26)

Carla is rarely mentioned in the book although it appears that the children spoke mostly Spanish together at home. There are a few comparative details noted by the father – Mario understood that he had two distinct languages at age two years and eight months, while Carla understood this concept three months earlier than her brother. Unfortunately we do not know much about Carla's speech, but we can assume that the two children would have jointly benefited from the Latino home environment, and Carla would have absorbed a great deal of language by listening and talking to her older brother.

The Saunders family: A dedicated father

George Saunders (*Bilingual Children: From Birth to Teens*, 1988) echoes the long-term studies by Werner Leopold and Alvino Fantini, except for the fact that the father spoke his second language. George, an Australian native, decided to speak his fluent second-language, German, to his children and the mother spoke only English (although she did understand some German). George Saunders described over 10 years of family interactions between the parents and their three children, Frank, Thomas and Katrina. They followed the OPOL strategy. Justifying his reasons for speaking in a second language to his children, George Saunders commented that as the sole German speaker in the family he felt '... the need for a regular conversation partner willing to talk only German with me at all times and on all topics'. George hoped that the family

---

George Saunders

Bilingual Children: From Birth to Teens 1988

Biographical data on children, Frank, Thomas, Katrina
From birth to adolescence

Mother – English
Father – English, German
Family living in Australia

Strategy: Non-native OPOL (German)

would have a chance to live in Germany on sabbatical, a goal which was achieved and the children were able to attend school in Germany.

Each child had its own allegiance to each language, with only the first child, Frank, feeling 100% bilingual. The children had small differences of ability. For example, at age three Frank was speaking German fluently with his father. Katrina spoke both languages when she was two years and six months, and it took Thomas until he was three years and nine months to feel comfortable in both languages. George concluded,

> ... even when growing up in the same family under basically the same conditions, children do not necessarily acquire bilingualism in exactly the same way. (Saunders, 1988: 96)

Despite only having their father speaking his second language and living in a monolingual community the Saunders children all became bilingual. This was remarkable, considering the lack of support in the community where they lived. The family had a strong sense of solidarity with the father's goal of bilingualism, even when faced with critical family, doctors and teachers. The children were able to tell stories and joke in the German language, thus achieving the father's goal of linguistic companions at home. The children often switched from German to English or vice versa, especially when retelling stories which involved a punch line or quotation in the language it referred to. The two boys generally used English together, except when they were playing a game with their father in German. They enjoyed having a 'secret' language which few Australians understand. English had an important place in the family too, as George acknowledged,

> That English is the language predominately used, even in private, between Thomas, Frank and Katrina, is a situation which has developed naturally, that is, practically without parental intervention. (Saunders, 1988: 61)

The Taeschner family: Wie bitte?

Professor Traute Taeschner (*The Sun is Feminine: A Study on Language Acquisition in Childhood*, 1983) documented the language development of her two German/Italian daughters from their first words up to age eight and nine. In the curiously titled book Traute focused on the early syntactical speech development of Lisa and her younger sister, Guila. The tape-recordings recorded lively exchanges between the two girls who were close in age and spent a lot of time together, and their mother who wanted them to speak only proper German with her. As the sole German speaker in an Italian environment, strictly following the OPOL approach, the mother disliked the girls speaking Italian to her.

Traute tried hard to keep the girls on track, refusing to reply when they used the 'wrong' language (Italian) with her. She subsequently applied the *Wie?* Strategy (translated as 'What did you say?') which forced the girls to rephrase a request in German if they wanted her to reply. Traute observed that her daughters unconsciously spoke

German together to get her attention, or to show Italians that they were bilingual. When they pretended to be their parents the 'mother' always spoke German and the 'father' Italian. Traute also reported several amusing anecdotes of the girl's refusal to accept that an object can have two names. Lisa and Guila's use of German together certainly benefited the family. Traute's daughters followed similar patterns of linguistic development, probably due to the fact that they were the same gender, close-in-age and enjoyed using language in their games together.

> **Traute Taeschner**
>
> *The Sun is Feminine*
> 1983
>
> Biographical data on her daughters Lisa and Guila
> From age 18 mths – 8 yrs and 1yr – 9 yrs
>
> Mother – German
> Father – Italian
> Family living in Italy
>
> Strategy: OPOL

Lisa and Guilia loved to play with languages and created an imaginary world called *Caratei* when they were six and seven years old. They chose a German-influenced name, but made it clear that it would be pronounced differently in Italian. Here is an extract of the description Lisa gave,

> I Caratei vivone su una nuvola e stanno così lontani che vedono la terre piccolo come un punto e le stele non le vedono neanche: Questo mondo si chiama **Schwighit** e si parla **Auet**. Gli italiaini dicone **Auèti**, ma è **Auet**. Per arrivare a quel mondo basta saper volare. (Taeschner, 1983: 224)

(The Caratei live on a cloud, flying and they are so far away that the earth looks like a dot and they don't even see the stars. This world is called Schwight and they speak Auet. The Italians call it Auèti, but it's called Auet. To get to that world, all you have to do is know how to fly.)

The Trilingual Hoffmann family

Professor Charlotte Hoffmann (*Trilingualism in Family, School and Community*, 2003) is Reader in Sociolinguistics at the University of Salford. Charlotte is German and her husband Spanish. In 1985 she wrote a fascinating academic paper about her two young German/Spanish/English trilingual children, Christina and Pascual. The family moved to live in England

> **Charlotte Hoffmann**
>
> 'Language acquisition in two trilingual children.'
> *Journal of Multilingual and Multicultural Development*
> 6 (6), pages 479–495. 1985
>
> Eight years of notes, diary entries and some tests on children, Christina (8) and Pascual (5)
>
> Mother – German/English
> Father – Spanish/English
> Family living in UK
>
> Strategy: OPOL + 1 (English from community)

when Christina was three years old. They followed a OPOL + 1 strategy, with English being the language of school and community. The issue was how Charlotte could maintain the two parental languages in a typically monolingual country. The family was able to employ German and Spanish au pairs to support the parental language acquisition. When Pascaul was born Charlotte asked her daughter, Christina, to speak German with him. The siblings established a bond with the language, and Pascual was motivated to speak German with his sister. Charlotte thought the children's different personalities affected their language use. Christina was described as 'more sensitive, thoughtful and reserved', while Pascual was more of an extrovert and was 'keen to establish contact with new people'. English sneaked into the siblings language use via the children's friends, as Charlotte observed,

> From an early age Pascual had some contact with English, first indirectly (television, listening to his sister play and talk with English children, etc.), and then from about the age of two more directly when he started to join in Christina's play more actively. (Hoffmann, 1985: 485)

The dominant language of the siblings soon switched to English as their 'preferred' language, when they began English-language schooling. Charlotte remarked that having two or more children in a family increases the contact with the outside language, although it can be beneficial for the younger one, who is able to practice with another child.

The Jisa family: Mixing in California

Harriet Jisa, from University of Lyon, France, studied the mixing patterns of her two young English/French daughters Odessa and Tiffany. The American mother and French father lived in France and the girls went to a local French preschool. They followed an OPOL strategy. Like Traute Taeschner's daughters, their dominant language was the country language and they were close in age. Harriet reported on a two-month stay the girls spent in California with their grandmother.

After an initial 'linguistic shock', on suddenly being immersed in a monolingual English-speaking society the girls adjusted their language use. The girls mixed languages frequently, especially between themselves and with their mother, who spoke English to them, but understood and accepted French responses. The girls perfectly

---

Harriet Jisa

'Language mixing in the weaker language.'
Journal of Pragmatics 32, pages 1363–1386. 2000

Snapshot biographical study on Odessa, 3 yrs, 6 mths and Tiffany, 2 yrs, 3 mths

Mother – English (American)
Father – French
Family lives in France, study reports on 2 mth stay in USA

Strategy: OPOL

understood each other's mixed utterances and were surprised when other people did not. By the end of their stay, they were mixing significantly less with outsiders, but between themselves still used French/English blends.

Since the mother understood French, it seemed that the girls felt comfortable adding in French words to their conversations. Interestingly, there was a subtle change of balance in the family, as the mother changed from being the only source of English in France, to being the only person the girls could use some French within America. The choice of mixed language between Harriet and her daughters seemed to work and created a way of communicating during a sensitive phase of their life.

The Caldas family: Keeping French alive in America

Stephen Caldas (*Raising Bilingual-Biliterate Children in Monolingual Cultures*, 2006) is Professor of Educational Foundations and Leadership at the University of Louisiana. Stephen, an American native and his French-Canadian wife, Suzanne, made a 10-year case study of their three children. After starting with the OPOL strategy the family evolved to maintain French in America.

Like Alvino Fantini, Stephen chose to speak his wife's language and they followed a *minority-language-at-home* approach. The family lived in a bilingual community in Louisiana, where a dialect of French was spoken, and the children attended bilingual elementary schools. Stephen and Suzanne collected data on the children's speech at home, typically while the family ate together. Stephen explained why he chose the unusual choice of mealtimes for collecting data,

> **Stephen J. Caldas**
>
> *Raising Bilingual-Biliterate Children in Monolingual Cultures*
> 2006
>
> Biographical data on children, John and twins, Valerie and Stephanie
> From age 9/7 yrs to young adults
>
> Mother – French (Quebec)
> Father – English
> Family living in Louisana, USA
>
> Strategy: OPOL at first/Minority Language at Home (French)

Importantly, this is the sole context that remained constant for all five family members over the entire study period, regardless of which country we were in. Also, it is significant that there was no overt pressure on the children to speak any particular language in the home at the dinner table, as both parents are completely bilingual. (Caldas, 2006: 25)

Stephen complemented this data with teacher surveys of their children's proficiency in both languages and self-surveys of how bilingual/bicultural the children felt. Stephen and Suzanne were particularly concerned that their children should sound 'right', having an American Louisiana accent, and a Canadian Quebecois French accent. The children did succeed in this goal, and were able to easily fit in and sound like their peers in either country. The book reports specifically on their three children's linguistic experiences of moving from elementary school to high school, and going through adolescence. Stephen Caldas gives a particular insight into the adolescent bilingual child's mind. Pleasing the parents by being bilingual was a strong motivating factor when the children were young, but it did not carry much weight with adolescents.

In American high school, French suddenly became 'uncool' as the children became teenagers. Even though they spent all their summers in a French-speaking environment in Canada, the children felt more attached to their American peers and lifestyle. The older brother, John, went through a language rebellion first, abandoning French when he started High School and causing a sibling rift. The twin girls were attending a French immersion program and felt more 'French', while their brother was pro-America and anti-French. Stephen transcribed eight-year-old Valerie demanding that her brother *'Parlez français!!'* (Speak French!!), to which 10-year-old John angrily replied 'English! English! English!' Later on, the balance changed when the girls abandoned French temporarily when they started High School. The self-conscious teens needed to have their bilingualism validated by their peers, and when they felt being bilingual made them different they quickly switched to being monolingual.

The Cruz-Ferreira family: Multilingual in Singapore

University Lecturer, Madalena Cruz-Ferreira (*Three's a Crowd? Acquiring Portuguese in a Trilingual Environment*, 2006) wrote about the first 10 years of life with her three children. Madalena is Portuguese and her husband is Swedish and both parents are multilingual. Karin, Sofia and Mikael, were brought up in a trilingual environment. The family lived with their young children in Sweden, Portugal, Austria, Portugal and Hong Kong. The family has lived in Singapore for 14 years and follows the OPOL + 1 strategy. The three children have attended English-language schools. The children were initially bilingual and subsequently became a trilingual family, with English as their third language. The Cruz-Ferreira family had to support three languages simultaneously, while being far away from Portuguese and Swedish-speaking family.

The young siblings began using Portuguese together when they were at home with their mother. The children spoke Portuguese to their mother and Swedish to their father. Each language had a strong cultural attachment, even for the other parent. Madalena noted that she would use Swedish words to talk about events linked to the Swedish language or Sweden, and likewise the father would use Portuguese. English had an important role in the cultural

---

Madalena Cruz-Ferreira

Three's a Crowd? Acquiring Portuguese in a Trilingual Environment
2006

Biographical data on Karin, Sofia and Mickael

Mother – Portuguese
Father – Swedish
English from the community
Family lives in Singapore

Strategy: OPOL + 1

and social life of the family, as a *lingua franca* and a school language. Both parents communicated in English with the children when helping them with their homework. Madalena observed,

> … the children also had early exposure to English, from exchanges with English-speaking guests or from social gatherings involving Swedish and Portuguese relatives or friends, who used English to communicate among themselves. (Cruz-Ferreira, 2006: 31)

Over time the three siblings decided to switch from Portuguese to mainly English as their 'preferred' language. Now trilingual young adults the children have access to several cultures and can choose where they live or study.

LINGUISTS RESEARCHING BILINGUAL FAMILIES

Not all linguists have bilingual children or want to study their own children. Instead they observe and report on other bilingual families. This gives an outsider's view on family language patterns, and a distance from the intense parent–child relationship which could affect language use. A linguist usually studies a child in their home environment, establishing a close relationship with the parents over a period of time (usually one or two years). Regular and detailed recordings are made of day-to-day language interaction. The majority of studies on bilingual child language focus on one first-born child (see studies by Elizabeth Lanza, Margerat Deucher and Suzanne Quay, Annick De Houwer and Jurgen Meisel). Nevertheless, there are a few interesting international case studies which include siblings. Eve Gregory investigated sibling support at home in recently immigrated Bangladeshi, Arabic or Chinese-speaking families learning English as a second language in London. Victoria Obied conducted a similar literacy study on four sets of siblings within bilingual families in Portugal. Christine Helot focused on trilingual Irish/French families aiming to support the Gaelic language. Japanese researcher, Masayo Yamamoto, studied Japanese/English families, and in Australia Susanne Döpke recorded parents maintaining German as a heritage language.

Eve Gregory: Siblings scaffolding languages in urban London

Dr Eve Gregory (*Many Pathways to Literacy: Young Children Learning with Siblings: Grandparents, Peers and Communities*, 2004) is a researcher in the Educational Studies department of Goldsmiths College in London. She has worked with children of newly immigrated extended families from Bangladesh, and children in urban London. Two of her case studies on Bangladeshi children in London are of particular interest (see also the research done by Charmian Kenner (2004a, b) on biliteracy and bilingual children).

In the first 1998 study the seven Bangladeshi children were in Year 1 of the British education system (where intensive reading takes place). Most of them came from large families, like Akhlak who is the ninth child of 11 siblings. Their parents did not necessarily have a high level of English and the children risked being left behind

Eve Gregory (1998)

'Siblings as mediators of literacy in linguistic minority communities'
Language and Education, 12 (1),
   pages 33–54, 1998

7 Bangladeshi-speaking children aged
   around 6 years living in London, UK

Strategy: Minority Language at Home
   (Bangladeshi)

Eve Gregory (2001)

'Sisters and brothers as language and
   literacy teachers: Synergy between
   siblings playing and working together'
Journal of Early Childhood Literacy, 1 (3),
   pages 301–322, 2001

16 families – 8 Bangladeshi compared to
   8 British children living in
   London, UK, with the oldest child
   aged 9, 10 or 11

Strategy: Minority Language at Home
   (Bangladeshi)

because they lacked literacy skills at school. Eve expected a parent to help them at home, but found that it was often an older sibling who read to the younger one. The older sibling would frequently ask questions about the text, or ask the younger one to 'recite' or repeat back what he or she had just read. This contradicted with the class environment where repetition was not encouraged and the children had to guess what the story was about before starting. Eve concluded that the sibling support was more suited to the children's needs, and should be taken into account by the teachers.

Eve's wider-scale 2001 study compared London children with Bangladeshi children. The synergy in the title refers to the way the siblings benefited from role-playing or 'playing school'. The younger children were described as '… excellent pupils, polite and knowledgeable, anxious to provide accurate answers'. Eve commented,

… content is transposed almost exactly and older siblings adapted almost the exact voice of the teacher, using her expressions, accent and intonations. (Gregory, 2004: 317)

The older child was able to practice being the teacher, and the younger child was able to practice in a safe environment away from the pressure of school. The school role-playing game was taken very seriously in the Bangladeshi homes, where dual literacy was highly valued.

Victoria Obied: Supportive and unsupportive families in Portugal

Victoria Obied, from Goldsmiths College in London, examined the biliteracy of four sets of siblings in Portugal and how the siblings supported the other's language use. The children were exposed to both cultures through their mixed-marriage parents. Unusually, two of the four families had step-siblings or parents who had remarried. Portugal has a predominately oral culture, with an emphasis on verbal communication in daily life and Victoria contrasted this to more literate British culture. Like Eve Gregory, she focused on how the siblings helped to support or 'scaffold' the emerging bilingual reading and literacy skills at home. Unfortunately, Families 1 and 2 did not have supportive sibling relationships. In Family 1, Victoria observed that the language balance changed when the second child, Alexandre, starting talking, because of his '…reluctance to interact with either his older brother or mother in the minority language [English].' The English-speaking mother and bilingual older brother, Mario, tried to help Alexandre with his English literacy. However, Alexandre strongly identified with the local Portuguese culture. Alexandre preferred his father as a linguistic role model and had effectively rejected his mother's and brother's language.

In Family 2 nine-year-old Claudia and her younger brother Jorge were close in age. The bilingual mother spoke fluent Portuguese and in the home mixed her two languages, leading to criticism from the father for not speaking enough English to her children, and from the children for her mispronunciation. The mother tried to establish a regular time for English through bedtime stories, but the children 'create a barrier …. and instead of responding to the shared intimacy of shared reading in their mother's first language, try to impose their own linguistic preferences …' The mother was able to help the children in translating across the languages but remained unsure of how to inspire her children to use English with her, or together.

> **Victoria Obied**
>
> 'How do siblings shape the language environment in bilingual families?' *International Journal of Bilingual Education and Bilingualism*' 12 (6), pages 705–720, 2009
>
> Study on four families in Portugal, Strategies: Some OPOL, some Mixed
>
> Family 1. Marco, 13 and Alexandre, 9 (English mother/Portuguese father)
> Family 2. Claudia, 9 and Jorge, 6 (English/Portuguese)
> Family 3. Justin, 17, Janet, 16 and Martin, 11 (Scottish mother/Croatian-American father, now with a Dutch stepfather)
> Family 4. Patrick, 11 and Alison, 6. (Portuguese mother/Irish Father)

The other two families were more supportive. In Family 3 the Scottish mother was previously married to a Croatian/American, and now had a Dutch partner. The three teenagers, Martin, Janet, and Justin had a strong sense of shared identity and support for their multilingual blended family. The younger siblings profited from the older one's language models. In Family 4, eleven-year-old Patrick and his six-year-old sister, Alison, had a Portuguese mother and an Irish father who loved storytelling. A high value was given to the father's culture and language, and biculturalism and biliteracy had been established. Contrary to the Caldas family, where bilingualism became more challenging with age, Victoria found that the older siblings found a role as 'mediators of both languages', as she concluded,

> … siblings play an influential role in shaping the language environment in families and this influence may increase as the siblings reach adolescence and parental influence lessens. (Obied, 2009: 718)

Christine Helot: Gaelic in Ireland

Christine Helot, from the Marc Bloch University in Strasbourg, specializes in French bilingual educational policies. In a 1988 study Christine observed two French/Irish families living in Ireland, where English and Irish (Gaelic) are spoken. Both families had French mothers, and Irish fathers. Like in the Caldas family, French language use was closely linked to one or two month summer holidays in France with family. In Family 1, both parents spoke French until the older child was three, when the father reverted to English after establishing French. The first son learnt English at school and studied Irish as a school subject. The second son heard English from his father, and also attended an English school with Irish lessons. In this family, Christine found a strong link with location; the family language changed depending on where they were. Together the siblings spoke mostly English in Dublin, a mix of French/English while on their annual holiday with grandparents in France, and interestingly a mix of Irish/French when on holiday in Ireland in an Irish-only summer-school (where their father taught Irish).

Family 2, followed the OPOL approach, with the mother speaking mainly French and the father mainly Irish. English language came 'from the street' from age three onwards, when the children went outside to play with local kids. However, English was excluded from the home (they did not have a television at home). Family 2 chose an Irish-medium primary school for their children, and consequently had a strong French/Irish home culture. Together the brother and sister spoke mostly French, mixed with a little English and a little Irish at home. They kept the same mix while on holiday in France, and in the summer school in Ireland.

> **Christine Helot**
>
> 'Bringing up children in English, French and Irish: Two case studies.'
> *Language, Culture and Curriculum* 1 (3), pages 281–287, 1988
>
> Family 1 – Two boys age 13 and 8
> Family 2 – Boy/Girl age 9 and 7
>
> Mothers – French
> Fathers – Irish (Gaelic)/English
> Families living in Dublin, Ireland
>
> Strategy: OPOL, with some Minority Language at Home

Masayo Yamamoto: Bilingual families in Japan

Masayo Yamamoto (*Language Use in Interlingual Families: A Japanese-English Sociolinguistic Study*, 2001), is Professor of Bilingualism Studies at Kwansei Gakuin University in Japan. Masayo studied bilingual Japanese/English families in Japan to see if the parent's

> **Masayo Yamamoto**
>
> *Language Use in Interlingual Families: A Japanese-English Sociolinguistic Study* 2001
>
> Study of 118 Japanese/English families, with all participants living in Japan
>
> Strategy: Some OPOL/some Minority Language at Home

attitudes and perceptions of bilingualism affected their future outcome. Of the 118 families she questioned in her study, about two-thirds had two children and 15 families had three children. Unlike many studies, Masayo included 'language spoken between the siblings' as one of her factors of language choices made between parents and their first, second and third children. Commenting on the sibling question, Masayo said,

> Having siblings, especially older siblings, will increase the opportunities for (younger) children to be exposed to a language which is not spoken at home, that is, the language spoken at school and/or in the immediate community. (Yamamoto, 2001: 10)

Masayo found that often the older siblings were 'more proficient in English', while the younger ones were 'more Japanese-orientated'. The parents thought this was due to different personalities or the amount of exposure to each language. Some of the parents blamed the older sibling for bringing more of the majority (Japanese) language into the house, and thought it was a disadvantage to have a two or more children. Masayo also considered the role of the peer group important, and noted that having local (Japanese) friends might lower the chance of the bilingual children speaking English, or any other minority language. Most of the siblings chose Japanese as their preferred language of communication together. For children talking directly to their sibling, nearly 50% of their speech was in Japanese, while around 45% preferred to mix, and only a small number of sibling sets used English exclusively. Masayo Yamamoto concluded that it was the children who preferred to speak Japanese to each other and to their parents (even non-Japanese parents). Unless the whole household used only English at home the children were tempted to rely more on Japanese, and were at risk of having passive bilingualism or becoming monolingual.

Susanne Döpke: OPOL in Australia

Dr Susanne Döpke (*One Parent, One Language. An Interactional Approach*, 1992) worked at the University of Melbourne and Monash University in Australia, before setting up a consultancy in Speech Pathology for bilingual families. Susanne conducted a well-known case study on the viability of the OPOL approach. She studied six young English/German bilingual children in Australia with similar linguistic backgrounds. Of the six, Fiona and Keith were considered most

Susanne Döpke

One Parent, One Language. An Interactional Approach
1992

Study on six children in Australia

(1) Keith, 2;8 English/German
(2) Alice, 2;8 German/English
(3) Jacob, 2;8 German/English
(4) Agnes, 2;8 German/English
(5) Fiona, 2;4 German/English
(6) Trudy, 2;4 German/English

Strategy: OPOL

successful in their acquisition of German. Keith benefited from having a German father, who worked hard to increase his German knowledge, and Fiona had more contact with German-speakers than the others. Both Fiona and Keith benefited from parents who helped increase their vocabularies.

Susanne purposely chose first-borns for her study, and made no mention of siblings in the beginning of the study. However, in a follow-up visit four years later, she noticed that all six children now had younger siblings and that the siblings all spoke English together. The siblings in the families of Trudy and Alice had not acquired any German at all, while Agnes and Keith had brothers who 'learned to understand German, but did not speak it'. Jacob's sister mixed German and English at the age of four. One positive case was in Fiona's family, where her two younger siblings both became actively bilingual. Susanne found this low count of second-born bilinguals disappointing, as she said,

> In spite of the fact that four of the younger siblings heard their older brothers and sisters speak German to one of their parents for at least a couple of years, only one child became actively bilingual. (Döpke, 1992: 198)

Susanne Döpke discussed the differences between the short-lag siblings (up to two years) and long-lag (three years or more). A child closer in age to a sibling might be more likely to copy the older one's linguistic patterns. The children in her study all had long-lag siblings, so perhaps they had less chance of picking up German from their older siblings. Nevertheless, they had all heard German in the home, and their parents were very positive about bilingualism, so we would expect more of the younger siblings to have picked up some German.

ADVICE FOR PARENTS IN BOOKS FOR BILINGUAL FAMILIES

The books and articles I have mentioned in the first part of this chapter are mostly academic in nature and not always easy for the general reader to understand. When linguists discuss the finer points of grammar or speech production it can read like they are using another language. For this reason, several books aimed at parents have been published in the last 20 years. These books give a broader view of the issues surrounding child bilingualism. I have chosen six books which touch on the subject of family language issues and sibling relationships. Incidentally most of the authors are parents, with two or more bilingual children themselves, and their personal experience is evident in the books.

Growing Up with Two Languages

Una Cunningham-Andersson's (*Growing Up with Two Languages: A Practical Guide*, 1999/2004) book is a practical guide to the basics of bilingualism. Una gives several examples of her own experience with her four English/Swedish-speaking children ranging from preschool to secondary school age. Una noticed that although all her four children were brought up in similar circumstances they have all turned out to be different kinds of bilinguals. The one factor they had in common was that they were all dominant in English until they started preschool around age three, when Swedish took over as their strongest language. The four children usually use Swedish together. The second-born child, Anders, had the most aptitude for languages and was able to easily reach monolingual standards in both languages. The children all had different levels of language skills or preferences, as Una explained,

> **Una Cunningham-Andersson**
>
> *Growing Up With Two Languages*
> 1999/2004
>
> Some biographical data on her children:
> Leif, 12
> Anders, 10
> Patrik, 6
> Elisabeth, 4
>
> Mother – English
> Father – Swedish
> Family living in Sweden
>
> Strategy: OPOL

> Leif (12;0) and Elisabeth (4;5) mostly answer in the language in which they are addressed, although their English is heavily laced with Swedish words … Anders (10;3) is very particular about keeping the languages separate, sometimes asking for vocabulary before he starts speaking. Pat (6;5) speaks only Swedish, although he understands English as well as Swedish. (Cunningham-Andersson, 1999: 32)

Nevertheless, Una considers that her children make an effort to speak proper English to monolingual English speakers. Una added that although some parents may try to persuade their children not to talk together in a certain language, the choice is out of their hands and they should not interfere. Una also noticed that sometimes older children use the minority language with a younger sibling 'if they believe it might get better results'. An older sibling might choose a parental or country language to sound more authoritative, or to boss younger siblings around. Alternatively an older sibling might use the minority language because he thinks that the younger one will understand it better.

The Bilingual Family Handbook

Edith Harding and Philip Riley (*The Bilingual Family – A Handbook for Parents*, 1986/2003) concentrates on practical and sensible advice. The book has a wide range of case studies, with several describing families with two or more children. A typical pattern the authors found is that the

> **Edith Harding & Philip Riley**
>
> *The Bilingual Family – A Handbook for Parents*
> 1986/2003
>
> Some biographical data on the Riley family – Swedish/English/French

siblings use the language of their school and/or community together. Harding and Riley agree that many parents find a wide difference between first and second children, but whether that is due to the child's aptitude or their parenting is an open-ended issue.

One case study describes an English family living in France (Harding & Riley, 2003: 96) who struggled to keep their home English-speaking only. Nevertheless their two teenage children continued to speak French together at home 'when the parents are not present', although they did made an effort to speak English to their little sister. Another sibling case study (Harding & Riley, 2003: 110) tells of a Danish/English family who had great success with their first-born daughter, who switched languages fluently and impressed everyone. Her younger brother had some delay, waiting until he was six to utter some Danish words, although he clearly understood the language. His parents confessed that they 'exercised far more control over their daughter than they did their son'. They agree that not being strict about him speaking Danish at home was kind, but did not help him in the long run.

Raising Multilingual Children

> **Tracey Tokuhama-Espinosa**
>
> *Raising Multilingual Children*
> 2001
>
> Some biographical data on children, Natalie, 7, Gabriel, 5 and Mateo, 3
>
> Mother – English
> Father – Spanish
> Family living in French-speaking part of Switzerland
> Two oldest children at German school
>
> Strategy: OPOL & 1

Tracey Tokuhama-Espinosa (*Raising Multilingual Children: Foreign Language Acquisition and Children*, 2001) discussed family strategies and the neurological workings of the bilingual mind in her book. Tracey's multilingual family used four languages used on a daily basis – English from the mother, Spanish from the father, French in the community (Switzerland) and German at school (for two of the three children). On siblings Tracey noted that younger children had 'an increased number of verbal exchanges'. This gave the younger ones a wider vocabulary and the older child a chance to practice his or her language skills with someone on the same level, linguistically and culturally. Tracey comments,

> If a child is lucky enough to have a sibling he is generally, but not always, rewarded in the area of language development. (Tokuhama-Espinosa, 2001: 86)

In the insightful diary excerpts at the end of book, Tracey wrote about her personal experiences with her three children. Tracey recounted how her oldest child, Natalie, was very 'maternal' toward her siblings, and sometimes talked for her younger brothers. Natalie subsequently became the 'official translator' for the two boys and decided to speak English with them (thus, reducing the father's minority language of Spanish used at home). There were times when she questioned her investment in bilingualism; when her second child refused to talk or when the oldest one found starting a new school hard. Tracey felt she didn't have much time to talk to her second and third children when they were babies, but she thought that having brothers and sisters compensated in the long run. They provided role-modeling of social behavior and use of appropriate language, which was very useful when it came to code-switching. In terms of personality, Tracey thought that Natalie's 'fast-paced, chatty, social character' overshadowed the quieter second child, Gabriel, who had to shout to have his turn at speaking. The third child, Mateo, seemed to have benefited the most, joining a linguistically solid family, with established routines and strategies.

A Parents' and Teachers' Guide to Bilingualism

Colin Baker (*A Parents' and Teachers' Guide to Bilingualism*, 2007) is organized in sections with a question and answer format. The book begins with *Family* questions, raising issues such as the mother's role, what to do if parents don't agree and the extended family. The second section on *Language Development* has a wide range of questions on age, gender, intelligence and how bilingualism develops over time. The third part deals with *Problems*, such as children refusing to speak a language, mixing, speech delays or more serious linguistic conditions like autism. This section also covers identity, personality and how children cope with being part of two cultures. *Reading and Writing* discusses biliteracy, and how parents and teachers can help support these skills. Education defines the types of programs available to promote bilingualism, along with how parents and teachers can make the right decisions for our children, regarding their schooling and language needs.

> **Colin Baker**
>
> *A Parents' and Teachers' Guide To Bilingualism* (3rd Edition) 2007
>
> Questions and answer format. Written for parents bringing up children bilingually and for teachers who need more information on bilingualism.

On siblings, Colin made the valid point that when the second child arrives the 'language pattern' of the household is well established. Consequently, the second or following child, are most likely to follow their siblings' preference for each language. Colin also notes how the older child is a strong language role model for younger siblings, saying,

> Older siblings have more power and become influential language models. Thus, younger siblings are sometimes slightly slower in their bilingual language development partly because they are excluded from the more advanced language interaction between mother and older siblings, and partly through copying older siblings. Older siblings also may tend to answer for their younger brothers and sisters! (Baker, 2007: 55)

The Bilingual Edge

Kendall King and Alison Mackay's book *The Bilingual Edge: Why, When and How to Teach your Child a Second Language* is full of facts for parents intending to bring up their children bilingually. It follows a question and answer format, grouped into themes of *Why, When* and *How* to teach your child a second language. The book is aimed at monolingual

> **Kendall King & Alison Mackay**
>
> *The Bilingual Edge*
> 2007
>
> Questions and answer format. Written for parents bringing up children with two languages, especially those teaching a non-native or L2 language at home.

parents in America and families with a heritage language (e.g. Chinese, Polish or Spanish) that has links to their family. The parents want their child to learn a second language, and do this either through a bilingual educational program, or by the parents using the second language at home. The advice in the book is for parents with babies or young children who are unsure about how to start introducing a second language in the home or through school.

The authors cover 10 'myths' which are commonly heard about bilingualism, such as that only bilingual parents can raise bilingual children, or that mixing languages is a sign of confusion.

One myth concerns siblings in particular: *Myth #4: Children who are raised in the same family will have the same language skills as one another*. Kendall and Alison say that there is always going to be some kind of difference between brothers and sisters, according to their individual personality or their memory skills. Kendall and Alison also discuss birth order and the effect if might have on language learning, saying that both parents and the older siblings have a 'big impact' on the language environments of younger siblings. The authors' remark,

> First-born children are far more likely to speak their parents' language than second-or third-born children. (King & Mackay, 2007: 24)

This might be due to the first-born's increased one-to-one time with a parent and the fact that the older sibling brings in the majority language (in most cases, English) into the home. Even if the first-born gets more individual time with their parents the second-born is not necessarily left unattended, because he or she gains from useful conversational skills such as knowing,

> … how to interrupt and get everyone's attention and how to understand who people are talking about when they use pronouns like "he" and "she". (King & Mackay, 2007: 79)

Raising a Bilingual Child

Barbara Zuer-Pearson (*Raising a Bilingual Child*, 2008) gives information on establishing bilingualism in the home and clear comparisons of strategies and current research comparing mono-lingual children versus bilinguals. Barbara also wrote an important chapter on children who may have problems learning two languages because of speech impairment. She also discusses children who might not get speech therapy because their bilingualism is seen to be the problem. In a section on families Barbara notes that older siblings can be helpful and show a good language model. However, Barbara cautions,

> **Barbara Zuer-Pearson**
>
> *Raising a Bilingual Child*
> 2008
>
> Written for parents bringing up children with two languages, with emphasis on USA bilingual provision, case studies and wide variety of examples of one-parent families, adopted children and older children.

> More commonly, though, older siblings bring more of the majority language into the house. They have majority-language friends who come to play, and they know about TV shows, comics, and movies in the majority language that you might prefer to avoid. When children are small, you are the major source of outside materials for your children, but as they get older, the children themselves play a larger role in selecting what they read or view on TV and whom they will play with. (Zuer-Pearson, 2008: 133)

There are several testimonials of families, with a wide-ranging view of divorced, single parents and adopted children all discussed, giving a good example of real bilingual families in America.

SUMMARY

We can see from the range of meticulous and detailed studies, compiled by the linguists and academics in this chapter, that each bilingual or multilingual family has its own unique history and way of blending the languages. The studies show several themes, one being that the father can play a key role in encouraging and supporting bilingualism in the early years, as commented on in the Leopold, Fantini, Saunders and Caldas families. A linguistically prodigious first-born child, like Hildegard or Mario, can perhaps have an early advantage over their younger siblings. The transition from home to school can provoke a change in children's language use as they become more affected by the outside world, as seen in the Tokuhama-Espinosa and Cunningham-Andersson families. An older sibling, such as Charlotte Hoffmann's daughter, can unintentionally 'bring home' the majority language of the school and community and increase its use at home. We also see that siblings can have a close intense relationship with a sibling supported by shared minority language use, like the Traute girls and the Saunders trio. As parents and educators we can learn from their personal stories and experiences with bilingual families about how to best help children growing up in a dual-language environment.

In Chapter 2 we discuss the bilingual or multilingual family. Which parent speaks which language to the children? Which strategy does the family choose to support bilingual language use? We also look at common issues in bilingual families. How do parents adapt their strategies, deal with relocation, and fine-tune their language use in the home with two or more children? In these times of change the parents might need to adapt their language use, and increase or decrease their use of one language in the home. We hear from over a hundred bilingual and multilingual families who completed an online survey, and see how real-life families adjust and evolve their language use as they grow.

Further reading on bilingual families

Academic studies and books on bilingual children

Caldas, S.J. (2006) *Raising Bilingual-Biliterate Children in Monolingual Cultures*. Clevedon: Multilingual Matters.

Cruz-Ferreira, M. (2006) *Three's a Crowd: Acquiring Portuguese in a Trilingual Environment*. Clevedon: Multilingual Matters.

De Houwer, A. (1990) *The Acquisition of Two Languages from Birth: A Case Study*. Cambridge: Cambridge University Press.

Deucher, M. and Quay, S. (2000) *Bilingual Acquisition: Theoretical Implications of a Case Study*. Oxford: Oxford University Press.

Döpke, S. (1992) *One Parent, One Language. An Interactional Approach*. Amsterdam: John Benjamins.

Fantini, A.E. (1985) *Language Acquisition of a Bilingual Child*. Clevedon: Multilingual Matters.

Grammont, M. (1902) *Observations sur le langage des enfants*. Paris: Mélanges Meillet.

Gregory, E. (1998) Siblings as mediators of literacy in linguistic minority communities. *Language and Education* 12 (1), 33–54.

Gregory, E. (2001) Sisters and brothers as language and literacy teachers: Synergy between siblings. *The Journal of Early Childhood Literacy* 1 (3), 301–322.

Gregory, E., Long, S. and Volk, D. (2004) *Many Pathways to Literacy: Young Children Learning with Siblings: Grandparents, Peers and Communities*. London: Routledge.

Helot, C. (1988) Bringing up children in English, French and Irish: Two case studies. *Language, Culture and Curriculum* 1 (3), 281–287.

Hoffmann, C. (1985) Language acquisition in two trilingual children. *Journal of Multilingual and Multicultural Development* 6 (6), 479–495.

Hoffmann, C. and Ystma, J. (eds) (2003) *Trilingualism in Family, School and Community*. Clevedon: Multilingual Matters.

Jisa, H. (2000) Language mixing in the weaker language. *The Journal of Pragmatics* 32, 1363–1386.

Kenner, C. (2004a) *Becoming Biliterate: Young Children Learning Different Writing Systems*. Stoke-on-Trent: Trentham Books.

Kenner, C. (2004b) Cantonese and Arabic-speaking pupils re-interpret their knowledge for primary school peers. In E. Gregory, D. Volk and S. Long (eds) *Many Pathways to Literacy*. Routledge: London.

Lanza, E. (1997) *Language Mixing in Infant Bilingualism: A Sociolinguistic Perspective*. Oxford: Oxford University Press.

Leopold, W.F. (1939, 1947, 1949a, 1949b) *Speech Development of a Bilingual Child: A Linguists Record* (in four parts). Evanston: Northwestern Press.

Obied, V. (2009) How do siblings shape the language environment in bilingual families? *International Journal of Bilingual Education and Bilingualism* 12 (6), 705–720.

Ronjat, J. (1913) *Le développment du langage observé chez un enfant bilingue*. Paris: Champion.

Saunders, G. (1988) *Bilingual Children: From Birth to Teens*. Clevedon: Multilingual Matters.

Taeschner, T. (1983) *The Sun is Feminine: A Study on Language Acquisition in Childhood*. Berlin: Springer-Verlag.

Yamamoto, M. (2001) *Language Use in Interlingual Families: A Japanese-English Sociolinguistic Study*. Clevedon: Multilingual Matters.

Guidance for bilingual families

Arnberg, L. (1987) *Raising Children Bilingually: The Pre-School Years*. Clevedon: Multilingual Matters.

Baker, C. (2007) *A Parents' and Teachers' Guide to Bilingualism* (3rd edn). Clevedon: Multilingual Matters.

Cunningham-Andersson, U. and Andersson, S. (1999/2004) *Growing Up with Two Languages: A Practical Guide*. London: Routledge.

Harding, E. and Riley, P. (1986/2003) *The Bilingual Family – A Handbook for Parents*. Cambridge: Cambridge University Press.

King, K. and Mackay, A. (2007) *The Bilingual Edge: Why, When and How to Teach your Child a Second Language*. New York: Harper Collins.

Tokuhama-Espinosa, T. (2001) *Raising Multilingual Children: Foreign Language Acquisition and Children*. Westport, CT: Bergin & Garvey.

Zuer-Pearson, B. (2008) *Raising a Bilingual Child*. New York: Living Language/Random House.

Chapter 2
The Growing and Evolving Family

I asked the families who participated in my survey about their choice of strategies and how they evolved over time. How did each family organize language use between parents, children and siblings? Some families had adapted their strategies over time, either becoming stricter, or more relaxed about controlling language use in the home. The birth of a second, third or fourth child could change language use. Parents reassessed or fine-tuned their strategies to suit the needs of more family members. Relocation was also a catalyst for changing strategies. A move to live in a different country, or a change of school language, could affect the language balance in the home. Siblings bringing home friends from school to play, who speak only the majority or country language could force a change of strategy within the family. The children became more vocal over time about which languages they thought their parents and siblings should speak. There were also some special situations where strategies had to be taken into account in line with the whole family's needs.

BALANCING MAJORITY AND MINORITY LANGUAGE USE

The language which is more dominant or widely used is often referred to as the *majority language*, and the less used language is the minority language. The majority language is usually the language of the community where the family lives and the *minority language* is linked to one or both parents. Each family has its own unique composition. Some families have one bilingual parent and one monolingual parent. In this scenario, one parent often does not understand or speak his or her partner's language. Some parents are both bilingual and switch from one language to the other with ease. There are families where three or four languages are used on a daily basis. Other families have parents who do not understand or speak each other's language, and who use a third language to communicate. Over time the balance can change; a monolingual partner might become bilingual. The couple may change the language they speak together. A move to live in another country might introduce a third language into the family. Language is a fluid and changeable entity and parents adapt along the way.

Throughout this book we hear about several academic case studies on bilingual and multilingual children alongside undocumented real-life stories of 22 families bringing up their children with two or more languages. One important piece of information we need to know is how does the family organize language use? Which language does the mother speak to her children? Which language does the father speak to his children? Which language do the parents speak to their children? What language do the children use to speak to each other? We also need to know how the languages exist in the home. Do family members mix languages or only use one language at a time? This information helps us build a picture of what is happening linguistically in the household. This description of language organization is known as the *Family Language Strategy*. Some strategies have names that are used in academic studies, such as *one parent one language (OPOL)* or *minority-language-at-home (mL@H)*. This coding of bilingual family characteristics is well established within the literature on bilingualism, and many parents writing on the internet forums or chatting in online forums on bilingualism use these codes to identify themselves as using a particular strategy. Naturally, not every family can be categorized and there are many variations on each theme. Here I have listed six types of family strategies, which have been documented in case studies and which we will be referred to in the book.

One-parent-one language (OPOL) – each parent uses their own language to the child
Minority-language-at-home (mL@H) – both parents speak the minority language at home
Non-native – one or both parents speak a second language to child
Mixed – two or three languages are used interchangeably
Trilingual – Lingua Franca – parents use a third language together
Time and Place – children learn second or third language in specific environment (i.e. school).

The strategies I discuss throughout the book are not always distinct and separate. In fact, many families overlap or combine two strategies. Families often begin with one strategy and adapt over time, for example, moving from OPOL to *minority-language-at-home*, to support the less-used language. The language use in the home is also different when parents are talking to a baby, a five-year-old child or a teenager. A strategy has to accommodate the linguistic options of each parent, in line with the language of the country and school.

Note: For a more comprehensive discussion on strategies see *Appendix 1 – Language Strategies*.

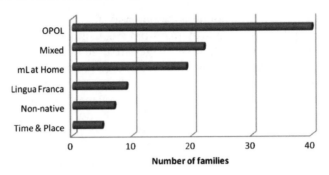

Figure 2.1 Strategies followed by families

I conducted an online survey on 105 international bilingual families and inter-viewed 22 families for this book (for more details see *Appendix 2 – The Online Survey*). The families were from all around the world and had two or more children. I asked the families to define the way each parent used languages within their family and to say which of the six strategies they considered themselves to be following at the time of the survey. One-hundred and two families responded to the question, and three families could not be classified in any category due to lack of information on inter-family language use (Figure 2.1).

The most popular strategy was OPOL with 40% of the 102 families following it. After OPOL, one in five families preferred a *mixed* language strategy, with 22% fami-lies choosing it, either with two or three languages. There were 19 families following *minority-language-at-home*, either parents who had the same nationality and first language and were living in a foreign country as expatriates or long-term immigrants or parents supporting a minority language at home. Parents using a third language between them, or the *Trilingual Lingua Franca* strategy accounted for nine families. There were seven families who were speaking their second or *Non-native* language to their children. Five families were following the *Time & Place* strategy.

> *Family language strategies* are dependent on the personal set of language skills, whether a parent can speak a partner's language and the language(s) of the coun-try where the family lives.

ADAPTING FAMILY STRATEGIES TO THE GROWING FAMILY

Does the arrival of another sibling affect the home language strategy? Would par-ents who used a strict strategy, such as *OPOL*, with their first child apply the same strategy to their second or third children or adapt to more relaxed strategy? I col-lected data on around a hundred international families using the OPOL approach (*Language Strategies for Bilingual Families: The One Parent One Language Approach*, 2004). These families showed a trend to adapt over time. Anecdotal evidence from parenting groups and web forums also suggests that many families started with a strict strategy and moved onto a mixed one with later-born children. Here is an example of how the bilingual family evolves as the family grows.

First child

The parents may do some research on bilingualism before their child is born, via websites, books or newsletters. They may choose a strategy straightaway, to suit their linguistic needs, or in the first year. Families might choose OPOL, mL@H or a mixed strategy depending on the parents' language level, location or preference for one strategy that a friend might have recommended. First-time parents are usually strict, and keen to justify their choice of strategy. They try hard to stick to the strategy, even when they are criticized by family or friends. Nevertheless, they may try out two or three different language strategies in the early years depending on how bilingualism is working out, or taking the advice of friends, family, doctors and teachers.

Second or middle child

The parents apply the same language strategy they had with the first child, especially if it worked well. Parents who decided to keep the same strategy were usually confident of their choice, and were better at ignoring any criticisms from teachers, family or friends. The parents might have found some friends with children who speak the minority languages, and with whom they can share cultural events together and increase minority language use in an informal way. Other parents may have found the strategy they used with their first child too strict, or just not suited to their overall needs. In the new circumstances, parents see that they may have even less time to talk one-to-one with each child and may decide to increase minority language at home. They may have moved house or changed the language of daycare or schooling for one child, bringing in more or less of one language into the home and changing the language balance.

Third or last child

Parents either stick with what has already worked with the other children of the family or adapt what they have leant to the new arrival. With the older siblings the parents may have slowly moved into using a more relaxed or mixed strategy, which relies more on the children deciding which language to use. Consequently a last child may try to copy the older sibling's speech patterns. Parents were usually not overly-concerned for a third child, unless he or she was not speaking well. They expect the older siblings to help out in a teaching role, by talking, singing or reading to the baby of the family.

Had any of the families I surveyed or interviewed changed strategies over time? Why did they change? Within the survey I asked them:

Have you changed your family language patterns after the birth of later born children?

Two-thirds of the families (68%) had not changed their strategy at all. One-third (32%) of the multilingual families had adjusted strategies along the way. I asked these families and the 22 case-study families to briefly explain why they had decided to change. Moving house or country was a frequent factor. Several families mentioned that their children were born in different countries, due to the families moving for work, to be closer to family or to increase exposure to one language. A change in the country language can mean that one or both parents have to adjust their strategy to suit the new linguistic situation. For example, a family with a Czech mother struggling to speak German in her German husband's home country then moved back to Prague where her language was spoken. With the children now benefiting from school, local activities and grandparents close by speaking Czech to their children, she chose to speak German more at home to support her husband. Important stages like the arrival of a new baby, a child starting school or becoming an adolescent can also affect the choice of strategy, and its success.

> **68%** of the families had not changed their language strategies
>
> **32%** had changed their strategy.

Two of the case study mothers, Christina and Martine, commented on sticking with the same strategy:

OPOL worked exceptionally well for our situation and was really the only option available since my husband is not that proficient in English and would have felt uncomfortable speaking to the children in a non-native language. We were very strict in using OPOL both inside and outside the house, no matter who was present, and it has paid off. My kids did change from speaking exclusively English with each other when they were very small to German as they got into school. That didn't change our OPOL plan, though.
Christina: English/German in Germany (OPOL), mother of Tom (15) and John (12)

You should never change your strategy – stability, perseverance and continuity give a good foundation. The child has to find its own space and has to evolve within a routine. By changing the strategy, I think that he might get lost or confused. Unless there is a medical problem such as delayed speech or any pathological problems diagnosed by a specialist, I do not think it is wise to change strategy.
Martine: French/English in Switzerland (OPOL), mother of Tiéphaine (9) and Xavier (7)

Some families said that they changed strategies because their experience with their first child had not been a success. With the second child they tried to either be more consistent in their home language use, or to be less strict, depending on the first or second child's reactions. The decision to apply the same strategy with a second child depended very much on how the first child reacted to the parent's initial choice, if it worked they probably will keep going as before, if not they might reassess and consider what they can do to help encourage bilingualism within the family. Several families in the study mentioned that having a second child was a point of reflection and a time when they could adjust or rebalance language use within the family. In the same way we might find our second child reacts in a different way to eating, sleeping or playing, we should consider that a second child may not accept language learning in the same way as the first one did. Forcing a child to communicate in a certain way may backfire in the long run, and what worked for the first one does not always work for the following children.

> Language use in the family *changes* and evolves as the family grows.

FINE-TUNING FAMILY LANGUAGE STRATEGIES

We now sprinkle more English into the home, whereas when we just had our first child we were more exclusive to Spanish

Often a new dynamic of language use between the children appears, pushing parent-orientated 'stricter' strategies out to a more child-centered and mixed way of communicating. Some strategies such as OPOL or *minority-language-at-home* demand that parents practice an essentially monolingual language use with their children. Parents can find it harder to pretend to two or more children that they do not understand the other parents' language, or will not speak a majority or country language with them. A trio of two adults talking directly to one child is often a success, because the child wants to communicate with his or her parents, and please them. The first child often does not realize that one or both of his parents could actually speak the other language. In fact the success of OPOL and minority language at home strategies rests on the basis that the child *has* to speak only one language otherwise the parent will not understand or reply. Having a sibling can dilute the intense one-to-one parent–child relationship, and some parents found they could not play the game of 'not understanding' one language with two children involved. Age differences can play a role as an older child knows the language abilities of the parents. One parent might decide it is not worth pretending he or she does not speak one language, knowing that the older one will tell the little one sooner or later.

As the older children start school and have a wider circle of friends and activities the language of the community becomes difficult to ignore or ban. Children began to have a say in language use, sometimes preferring to speak a different language to what the parents chose. Parents may be less serious about policing language use at home and allowing exterior or nonparental language use at home. Parents also noted that it was harder to control the language the siblings choose to use together, especially when they played together, away from the parents, and created their own mixes and interlanguage translations. Mixing also increased as siblings found their own way to communicate with two languages, and likewise, parents might find themselves unintentionally mixing more in their daily speech too. There were also some families who adapted their strategies to suit circumstances that they had not expected, like a child who had speech problems, emotional problems caused by moving to live in a country with a new language, or introducing new family members like a stepmother or stepsiblings with different language needs. All these reasons can influence a family language strategy and whether it works or not.

There are many areas open for discussion in the family home. When should the 'other' language be used? How strict should parents be about using the 'wrong' language or lazy translations? Should parents pick up on words or phrases that are commonly mistranslated and correct sloppy language use? What if you want to tell your family about something closely linked to one language and need to switch into the other language? One issue many parents agreed on was that when children begin formal schooling the parents could not avoid doing homework in the 'other' language. Madelana Cruz-Ferreira, linguist and mother of three Portuguese/Swedish/English trilingual children, commented on the difficulties of remaining loyal to your own language (personal communication, January 2008):

> Like many self-labelled so-called 'OPOL' parents, we found ourselves using all three languages in our family. For example, I use my second language (Swedish) words/expressions to talk about Swedish-bound happenings, memories, etc. Their father does the same in Portuguese for the same reasons, and both of us used English to discuss school homework when the children were small.

Here are some comments by case-study parents, Odile and Tammy, on the subtle changes in language use, created by homework and outside events.

> *Since having children we stuck to Dad speaking English and Mum French and it seems to work. My husband and I speak French at home, but the children always address him in English. The one thing I make allowance on is when Amy and I do Maths homework [she attends an English language school], and I will say some numbers in English because I realized she was confused with the French numbers. If the children get lazy with me and start introducing shorter English words or bad English translations into our conversations, I'm very strict in the sense that I make them repeat the correct word or sentence in French.*
> Odile: French/English in Malaysia (OPOL), mother of Amy (7), Luca (5) and Elliot (1)

> *We are bringing up our children using our second language (Spanish) at home. Between us we felt more comfortable speaking English to each other since our Spanish level is 'conversational' and at an elementary level. Our oldest daughter, Isabel, quickly surpassed*

our Spanish level threshold when she was around six or seven years old. When she started elementary schooling it became difficult for us to discuss certain concepts with her in Spanish, like religion, nature and all those Why? questions children of that age ask their parents. We simply had to reply in English.
Tammy: English/Spanish in the United Kingdom (mL@H), mother of Isabel (8), Elena (6), Monica (3) and Nora (1)

RELOCATING AND REBALANCING LANGUAGE USE

We switched country of residence, and added the grandparents into the picture

Moving house and changing the country language can be one reason why parents have to adapt language use in the home. In my survey, nearly half the families had lived in their country for over 10 years. Other families had lived in two or more countries over the last 10 years though, and some of the siblings were born in different countries. Many bilingual families moved house every two or four years. This was usually for a parent's job or a return to a parental country after time away. A move to a country where a different language was spoken often put the parent's choice of language strategy into question. With a new community language, and perhaps a new school language too, the dominant language of the home could rapidly change over a few months. These changes could destabilize the family language strategy and needed adjustment.

- 17% of the families had lived in their current country of residence for 1 to 3 years.

- 18% from 3 to 5 years.

- 25% had been there from 5 to 10 years.

- 40% were long-term residents, 10+ years.

Some children had emotional reactions to the changing languages and needed extra support as some of the case-study mothers reported. One mother home-schooled her son for a year until she felt he was ready for the wider world of the local school. Parents in a trilingual family dropped down to two languages with a change of country, while others suddenly found themselves in a trilingual situation. Other families benefitted from an increase in language support from extended family living nearby. A new school was able to support a minority language and take the pressure off the parents.

Here are two examples from three mothers, Alice, Andrea and Josie, who experienced changing countries and language strategies. First, Alice describes how her trilingual family dealt with a move from Spanish-speaking environment to a Germanic one, and how they resolved the problem of finding a place for English in their new home.

After our daughter was born, we lived in Ecuador and decided to use the OPOL method (with me speaking German and my husband Spanish). We kept English for communication between ourselves. This worked very well for as long as we lived in Ecuador. Then we decided to move to Austria, where the majority language is German. We stuck to our OPOL method for two years, until I realized that my daughter was overexposed to German. She got German from kindergarten and then all day from me as well. English and Spanish she'd hear only after her father got home from work in the evening, for a few hours. Even though it was clear that she understood English and Spanish, she would reply only in German. This frustrated my husband, who, with his limited German skills at that time, felt he could not really communicate with Isabella.

We decided to switch to another model: minority-language-at-home. The plan was to reinforce English by declaring it a family language, meaning at home we always speak English with everyone, also to the kids. We left German to the environment and the grandmother, and my husband still spoke Spanish when interacting on a one-on-one basis with the children. So what we have now is a bit of both models: minority-language-at-home with OPOL (used mainly by my husband). We expected all sorts of problems, but surprisingly, my daughter reacted very well to this change. She actually seemed to like the fact that we also spoke English with her directly. This helped her activate English and we could include her in our conversations. Two years later, she converses in English with both of us, as well as with her little brother. She even insists that I speak English with her in the presence of her German-speaking friends when I pick her up from Kindergarten.

Alice: German/Spanish/English in Austria (lingua franca), mother of Isabella (5) and Dominik (2)

German mother Andrea had lived in Britain for nine years where she supported German in an English-dominated environment with her seven-year-old daughter from her first marriage. After returning to Munich with her second husband, and the birth of two more children, the language strategy was reversed and Andrea supported English at home now.

In Britain, I spoke German to Melanie with a strict language strategy at young age (For example, I would say, in German "I don't understand" when Melanie would speak English to me). After moving to Germany, we decided to speak English to keep practicing it. I stuck to that even when Melanie's language use became more and more German. Rainer always spoke German with Melanie and she with him too.

When Lena was born in 2001, a decision as to language use in the family was taken. In order for Lena to grow up bilingually too, the home language would be English. Melanie was told to speak in English to Lena and thus help her learn to speak English and teach her. The same applied when Finlay was born. If Lena spoke German to Finlay, I would point it out and say that she should speak English since otherwise Finlay would not learn to speak English properly. Lena used English until she was three and a half years old.

After about 6 months in Kindergarten she would answer in German. Lena now speaks German to her parents, however, she still speaks English with her brother.
Andrea: English/German in Germany (L2 at H), mother of Melanie (15), Lena (6) and Finlay (3)

IN COMES THE MAJORITY, OUT GOES THE MINORITY

We speak more English since our first child has started school in England

Marjukka Grover, editor of *The Bilingual Family Newsletter* wrote about her personal experience with her two Finnish/English sons, and being a mother speaking a minority language, Finnish, in England, as she observed in a 2005 article:

> When a child joins a majority language nursery or playgroup the parents will get some idea of how powerful the majority language can be. However, it is not until formal schooling starts that the full force of this process becomes apparent. Some families are lucky to live near an International School, but most children will enter into the local majority-language school system and may become embarrassed to speak a language that other children don't understand. (Grover, 2005: 1)

Parents often remarked that when an older sibling brought friends from kindergarten or school or the neighborhood home to play the siblings chose to speak the language of the country, school or the majority language. Younger siblings liked to copy older siblings. This was a testing time for families following OPOL, *minority-language-at-home* or *non-native* strategies, who tried hard to use only the minority language at home, and limit the majority language to school or outside the home. The local children who came to play would naturally choose to watch television in the majority language or play games using the majority language. The parents of small children agreed that when friends came to play it was important that everyone understood each other, and that the invited children did not feel excluded linguistically. Consequently, a minority-language parent might use the majority language with the invited child or translate everything and even speak the majority language with their own children.

Siblings are aware of these subtle changes in family language interactions and a younger sibling could quickly pick up the message that the minority language is not worth much, or that it is not necessary to learn it since the local kids only speak the majority language. A younger sibling might decide not to speak the majority language to both parents, since they clearly understand it. This can destabilize a strategy, like *minority-language-at-home* or OPOL, because parents speak less and less to their children in the minority language. Here are comments from case-study mothers, Lilian, Theresa and Josie on how the majority language can slowly suppress minority language use.

Our strategy is speaking the minority-language-at-home. However, since our oldest son became fluent in English he sometimes speaks English to us, and, without thinking about it, we reply. Or once in a while we have to speak English while helping him with homework.
Lilian: English/Portuguese in the United States (mL@H), mother of Kelvin (5) and Linton (3)

When my husband and I met we spoke only in English, but after moving to Spain we started using more and more Spanish. With our eldest daughter, we started speaking only in English, but when she started playing with other kids and going to school, we began using more Spanish. Since the kids speak in Spanish to each other, our conversations often switch over to Spanish too.
Theresa: English/Spanish in Spain (OPOL), mother of Carmen (13), Rocio (11) and Violeta (9)

Malaysian mother Josie lived in Singapore before, with her children attending a German-language school. When she returned to live in her husband's country, Germany, she found it hard to keep English on the agenda.

When we lived in Singapore, we encouraged the children to speak German to each other, although being at the German School they were never in the danger of forgetting the language. We tried to reverse that after returning to Germany, but the children cannot be persuaded to speak English between themselves. Only Lukas, who is 4, will sometimes still say something to his brothers in English, but that is increasingly rare. In view of the fact that Tobias was (and still is having problems speaking English) we have even tried insisting that the language spoken by all of us – including my husband – when we are together should be English, but to no avail. Any attempt at this lasts about two minutes before everyone goes back to German. My husband and I continue to speak our own languages to the boys, only making an exception out of politeness when we are in the company of people who would not otherwise understand what we are saying.
Josie: Chinese/German/English trilingual family in Germany, mother of Niklas (12), Tobias (8) and Lukas (4)

SPECIAL SITUATIONS

With my son, we were 100% OPOL, but because of my son's refusal to speak French, I started to speak some French within the family, for example, joining in when my partner had started a conversation in French

In some families there was sometimes a more specific reason for changing or adapting strategies within the family. This could be due to one child's refusal to speak one language, or a delicate linguistic situation such as when an adopted, foster or step-child joined the family. It could also be a linked to a teacher or speech therapist who recommends 'dropping' one language for the good of the child. All these sensitive issues needed careful thought from the parents on how to accommodate the needs of one or more child within the whole family. Here two case-study mothers, Gerry and Jenifer, describe how special circumstances in the family meant family strategies were adapted for their children. Gerry, mother of four English/Spanish-speaking children, comments on the family decision to drop OPOL for a while to help their third son gain some confidence in English in Canada. Both parents spoke English, although the father still spoke Spanish to the other siblings. After a subsequent move to Mexico the parents then chose to home-school the third son for a year to help him settle into his new Spanish-speaking environment.

> We had one son (our third born) who was speech delayed and so my husband began to use only one language (English) with him. Our language of major communication at the time was English at home, but the older boys were in French immersion school and my husband had been speaking Spanish (his first language) with the boys at home. This lasted until our third born son began to use English well and had a firmer grasp on it. Then we went back to the OPOL method to integrate more Spanish into his daily listening and verbal communications.
>
> When we went back to Mexico, the same son had a minor emotional crisis upon being immersed into the Spanish school environment, so I home-schooled him for almost one year until he had a firmer grasp on Spanish, which was then the language of major communication in society and at school. He did very well afterwards and mastered his second language to the degree that he was first place in a class of 33 students (in grade 1) last year.
> Gerry: English/Spanish, now living in Canada, mother of four children (aged 13, 11, 7 and 5)

Jenifer and her husband have adopted three children. As fluent speakers of Japanese as a second language they have lived in Japan twice. Jenifer decided to speak Japanese to Lachlan when he was two years old and has continued with the two younger siblings.

> My oldest son, Lachlan, came to Japan with my husband and I when he was three months old. I didn't really have to make the decision to speak Japanese to him since he was getting enough input in his Japanese daycare. So when we got back to the US [when he was 18 months old] I was speaking some English and then kind of translating into Japanese. He was about 2 when I made the decision to speak to him entirely in Japanese.
>
> Our second child, Kiki, was born in Japan and when we adopted her, at age one, I told the Child Welfare Office I would speak Japanese to her. It became less of just a game and more a feeling that I could help her retain her ethnic identity so that if she ever wanted to return to Japan to live she could. And we kept returning to Japan, which made it easy to keep it up.
> Jenifer: Japanese/English in USA (L2 at H), mother of Lachlan (9), Kiki (5) and Case Kaye (1)

THE FIRST OR ONLY CHILD

With one child we can control what language he speaks at home

The majority of the recognized academic studies and texts on bilingual children, published over the last century, have focused on only children or first-borns as we discussed in Chapter 1. The first-borns may have a younger brother or sister in the background, like Hildegard Leopold or Mario Fantini, but the younger siblings are rarely taken into consideration. This type of 'first-born/only-child' case study was well suited to analyzing speech data on parent–child speech. There may also be another factor that parents with one child are perhaps keener to participate in academic case studies than those with larger families The only or first child often has their parent's undivided attention, at least until a second child arrives. An only child can be keen to please the parents and motivated to speak, read and write well. Parents with one child may benefit from more time with their child, and may be able to fine tune their language use to fit their child. Nevertheless, raising one child bilingually can be challenging. Parents often seem to be having a hard time struggling with bilingualism with their first or only child. A browse through internet chat rooms and bilingual parenting magazines shows that the majority of queries and questions are from first-time parents or those with one child. It seems more important to succeed and get it right with the first or only child. As one parent commented 'the not-knowing whether or not your child will become bilingual can be very stressful. There is a lot of pressure to get it right'.

Is it easier to establish and maintain bilingualism with just one child? This is a sensitive issue because we cannot fairly compare one-child families against those with two or more children. There are families who have one child now, but may have more children in the near future, and families who only have one child by choice or because they cannot have any other children. Each family has its own choices to make about how many children they have. However, it is interesting to consider only children or the first child briefly because parents and children do appear to have a different experience of establishing and maintaining bilingualism in a triad of mother–father–child. It might appear to be easier to bring up one child bilingually because parents have more time to talk, listen and encourage their emerging dual language skills. Parents might be able lead conversations with their child to help them learn new vocabulary. They can pick up on language errors or gaps in the child's vocabulary quickly and react to their language needs. I asked parents to reflect on their experiences with their first child, before a second child arrived, and respond to the statement.

Establishing bilingualism is easier when you have only one child

In fact, only 18% of the parents (19 parents) thought it was easier with one child (Figure 2.2). Sixty-nine percent of parents (73 parents) disagreed with the statement, with a third of the parents disagreeing strongly. There were 13 parents who were undecided. The survey families were not convinced that only having one child was easier and any benefits of 'extra quality time' were overshadowed by sibling bonding

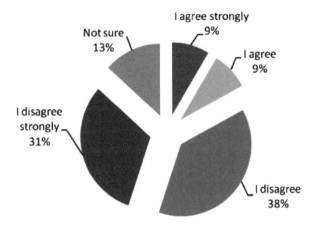

Figure 2.2 Establishing bilingualism is easier when you have only one child

and interaction. Nevertheless, parents were concerned that the first child had a different experience. For practical reasons some parents found that they did not have the same enthusiasm about language acquisition. One opinion frequently expressed in bilingual families is that the following siblings simply do not get the same level or quality of parental input that the first one did. This can mean the older child gets a solid knowledge of both languages, while other children learn a weaker version, from their siblings than their parents. This was especially true when things have gone well with the first child and bilingualism has been successfully established. Gerry, a mother of four children, speaks for many parents when she says her experience with one was special:

> *When I only had one child I spent all of my time talking to him and bathing him in my native language. Later, when I had more children my time and that level of enthusiasm and energy was diluted and divided among them. Exhausting! I did a lot of quiet gesturing and humming with subsequent children; and so, the language use they were exposed to was not on par with that of my first-born son (who began speaking at 6 months of age and has not stopped since).*
>
> Gerry: English/Spanish in Canada (OPOL), mother of four children (aged 13, 11, 7 and 5)

The tendency to focus on one-child families is important because these one-child studies are the basis of much of the advice given to parents regarding bilingualism. Since many of the studies on bilingual children report on young or preschool aged children, it perhaps falsely appears that the parents have 'succeeded', when the linguistic outcome of the child, five or 10 years later, could be very different. They are not misleading in any way, but we should be careful not to assume that what works in a one child scenario works in the rather messier and complicated larger group of a family with two or more children.

> What works with *one child* may not always work in a family with two or more children.

SUMMARY

This chapter shows the diversity of the ways bilingual and multilingual families operate. From each parent strictly using only one language, to parents who mix three languages all the time, there is no right or wrong way to organize language use in a bilingual family. Families might start with one strategy and find that their needs evolve over time. Strategies are also flexible and adaptable. Some changes in a child's life can precipitate language shifts. Families may find that moving house or changing countries can affect the language balance, especially if a new language is introduced or one language goes from majority status to minority. Children starting school and bringing home friends to play can also change the language use in the home, perhaps making the minority or less-used language more at risk of being passive. As they mature the children might have a preference for using a certain strategy at home and may put pressure on their parents to stop, start or mix languages, depending on the individual situation.

In the next chapter we look at emotional and practical side of the sibling relationship. The choices of language the siblings make independently of their parents. What criteria do siblings use for choosing a language they use together? Is it a parental language, a country language or a school language? Does the school language have a strong effect on the sibling's choice of language use together? Can siblings support and maintain a minority-language at home, giving one or both parents conversational partners and keeping it active? These issues are covered in Chapter 3.

Further reading on evolving families

OPOL

Barron-Hauwaert, S. (2004) *Language Strategies for Bilingual Families: The One Parent One Language Approach*. Clevedon: Multilingual Matters.

Caldas, S.J. (2006) *Raising Bilingual-Biliterate Children in Monolingual Cultures*. Clevedon: Multilingual Matters.

De Houwer, A. (1990) *The Acquisition of Two Languages from Birth: A Case Study*. Cambridge: Cambridge University Press.

Deucher, M. and Quay, S. (2000) *Bilingual Acquisition: Theoretical Implications of a Case Study*. Oxford: Oxford University Press.

Döpke, S. (1992) *One Parent, One Language. An Interactional Approach*. Amsterdam: John Benjamins.

Grover, M. (2005) The benefit of hindsight: The changing challenges of bilingual children. *The Bilingual Family Newsletter* 22 (4), 1–3.

Lanza, E. (1997) *Language Mixing in Infant Bilingualism: A Sociolinguistic Perspective*. Oxford: Oxford University Press.

Leopold, W.F. (1939, 1947, 1949a, 1949b) *Speech Development of a Bilingual Child: A Linguists Record* (in four parts). Evanston, IL: Northwestern Press.

Taeschner, T. (1983) *The Sun is Feminine: A Study on Language Acquisition in Childhood.* Berlin: Springer-Verlag.

Yamamoto, M. (2001) *Language Use in Interlingual Families: A Japanese-English Sociolinguistic Study.* Clevedon: Multilingual Matters.

Minority-language-at-home

Fantini, A.E. (1985) *Language Acquisition of a Bilingual Child.* Clevedon: Multilingual Matters.

Trilingual/multilingual

Hoffmann, C. (1985) Language acquisition in two trilingual children. *Journal of Multilingual and Multicultural Development* 6 (6), 479–95.

Tokuhama-Espinosa, T. (2001) *Raising Multilingual Children: Foreign Language Acquisition and Children.* Westport, CT: Bergin & Garvey.

Non-native

Saunders, G. (1988) *Bilingual Children: From Birth to Teens.* Clevedon: Multilingual Matters.

Time and place

King, K. and Mackay, A. (2007) *The Bilingual Edge: Why, When and How to Teach Your Child a Second Language.* New York: HarperCollins.

You can read more about the families of Christina, Martine, Alice, Andrea, Lilian, Theresa, Josie, Odile, Tammy, Gerry and Jenifer at the end of the book in *Family Profiles.*

Chapter 3
The Sibling Relationship

This chapter looks at the linguistic relationships siblings can have at home. We know a great deal about parent–child bilingual language use, but very little about which language siblings prefer to use together. Do the siblings prefer a parental language, a school language, a mixture of two or more languages or a language not used in the home? In most families it is the children who decide, not the parents. We look at the choices bilingual siblings make for their 'preferred' language. In theory, having a sibling who speaks the minority, or weaker parental language, to another sibling would be an advantage for the parents. This could help keep this language use active and fresh through the children's imaginative talk. Might siblings speaking the minority-language together be the key to maintaining it?

Throughout this chapter we consider some of the diary data and refer to the academic case studies on bilingual families, who were introduced in Chapter 1, along with comments from the bilingual and multilingual parents that I interviewed via the survey and case studies.

OUR 'PREFERRED' LANGUAGE

They chose which language they spoke together ... we had no say in it!

For our firstborn we could rigidly separate the languages we used. The second and third children they use more German at home. i.e. the environment language.

One of the most interesting factors of the bilingual family is the question of *which* language the siblings choose to communicate in. The common language the siblings choose to use together is often referred to in academic research as the *preferred* sibling language. It is their private language and can be one language or a mix of two languages. The choice is often subconscious, arising simply from a need for siblings to communicate effectively. The preferred language is the language that the siblings use to play, make up jokes, tell stories and argue in. This preferred language is used when the parents are not around, so it is not strictly necessary to use a parental language. Even if the parents do not approve or agree with the language selected, there is little they can do to control language use in such private contexts. The parents might have some influence in which language becomes the preferred one, but in the long term, it is the *children* who choose. The chosen language(s) must be accepted by all the siblings for it to work. In some cases children do speak different languages to each other, but this is usually temporary, for example, when one child starts school has more exposure to one language.

From the limited information we have, younger children appear to be guided by the older child, who sets the precedent. Case studies and data on families show that the siblings tend to use at least one parental language. If not, the default option is a school or country language. It can take time for siblings to find the best combination; they may prefer to stick with one language exclusively or mix two or more together. The choice also depends on the sibling's contact with the outside world, especially school and friends, who may have an influence on their language preference. A typical pattern is that the mother's language is the preferred language when the children are at home with her for most of the day. When school begins and the children find new friends from outside the home the peer group language has a stronger influence.

There is very little research on the language choice of siblings, probably because of the difficulty in obtaining detailed data on language use without a parent or researcher present. In classic observations of bilingual children the family language use transcribed is usually between the father or the mother and one child. The issue of child-to-child language use in a bilingual family has probably been under-estimated by researchers in the field. Data on unsupervised sibling-to-sibling language use is difficult to collect, simply because the recordings have to be done away from an adult. When a parent (or researcher) is present the siblings are tempted to adjust their speech to suit him or her accordingly, sometimes without even realizing it. Siblings can even change languages when a parent enters the room, without directly speaking to them. Asking the parents which language their children prefer can be biased, because a parent might answer that their children naturally prefer to speak their language. Nevertheless, most parents probably know which language their children use together when they are playing together. Ideally, researchers could hide recording devices in the areas where the children play, but this could pose ethical problems with regards to private conversations.

Being a parent *and* a linguist is one way around the problem of privacy. Stephen Caldas and Madalena Cruz-Ferreira compiled diary studies of their respective three children and unobtrusively recorded genuine family conversations either around the dinner table, or when their children were talking or playing games together and unaware they were being taped. In the Caldas family the sibling's preferred language changed as the children grew up. Stephen Caldas taped his family conversations while they ate together at the dinner table, and was able to regularly record his children's relatively natural language use over a long period and calculate the percentage of French and English as they chatted together. According to Caldas' diary entries, the children preferred French when they were young. They all attended bilingual schools and spent their summers with French-speaking family or in French-language camps in Quebec. However, as the oldest child, John, reached adolescence and started High School, he became significantly more Anglophone and refused to speak French at home, especially with his sisters. The lowest point was in May 1996, when John was 10 years old and Stephen counted 'zero' French words. The girls reacted badly to this change of sibling language, demanding of their brother to '*Parlez en francais!!*' This had little effect since John was simply more influenced by his new school friends than his young sisters. Two years later, the 10-year-old girls also began replacing French with English and copying their brother's linguistic choices. In one year their French conversation levels, around the dinner table, plummeted from roughly 95% French in the summer to about 25% by the September, when the girls started fifth grade. This was in spite of the fact that the twins were still attending a bilingual school. Here is an example of the family language use six months later,

> I videotaped at least half hour of Christmas morning interaction in 1997 when the twins were 10;7 and John was 12;7. There was much communication among all family members. Suzanne and I spoke some French, but the children spoke only English. (Caldas, 2006: 67)

The mutual decision to switch from French to English in the Caldas household took a few years to be resolved. By the time John was 15, and the twins were 13, all the family conversations recorded in America were in English. Despite the sibling switch to English when Stephen made recordings around the dinner table in Quebec the French levels peaked again. As Stephen sums up, it was not that the children could not speak both languages together, they simply chose *not* to. Caldas remarked perceptively,

> The children were exhibiting parallel monolingualism more than classic bilingualism. (Caldas, 2006: 68)

In trilingual families there are three options for the siblings preferred language. A pragmatic choice, based on their school and society, is often the best solution. Interestingly, in some trilingual or multilingual families neither parental language is chosen. The siblings often prefer a school language or country language. This is a logical choice as the children know they can all communicate in their lingua franca with friends and local children. Madalena Cruz-Ferreira observed how her three trilingual Portuguese/Swedish/English children changed their preferred language over time. In the early years, Portuguese (the mother's first language) was used, but the siblings evolved to prefer English. The family lived in Singapore, where English was frequently used at school and in the community; and the children attended

English-curriculum International schools. As Madalena says (personal communication, January 2008),

> Unlike Swedish, Portuguese had no support when the children grew up, except from me. Yet being 'mummy's language' (the parent who was also the main caregiver) made the children start using Portuguese among themselves, as their first peer language. The children's own institution of English as their own language in the family provided them with a peer bond that they wouldn't have been able to forge with either mum's or dad's language. It was this natural evolvement of language uses, of the children's own making, that made our family trilingual and not bilingual, as mum and dad had 'planned' in the first place.

Madalena noted that as teenagers the children had to reassess their preferred language again:

> When Karin moved to Sweden to study (aged 16), she naturally started addressing her siblings in Swedish, her new-found peer language. Sofia refused to respond in that language and used their usual English back to her sister. Mikael was more laid-back and just responded in whatever language he was addressed in. This Swedish 'intrusion' on their peer-language was short-lived, though. Karin lives in England now, Sofia and Mikael live in Sweden, and English still is their common language.

The sibling agreement on which language suits their needs is an important factor in preferred language use. Siblings may take time to 'sort out' which language suits them in their own circumstances and what works best for them. Since the preferred language is not tied to a parent's language the children have to each adjust their personal language preferences alongside their sibling's needs to find out which language feels more comfortable and 'right' for them. What works best for young children playing together with trains or dolls might not be the right option when they are preadolescents or teenagers, sharing music or watching films together. Sibling language preference can also be affected by external factors, such as the language of the country where they live, their school and friends.

> Bilingual siblings often have a *preferred* language that they use together. It could be a parental language, a school language, a community language or a mix of two or three languages. The preferred language can change over time and across contexts

CHILD-TO-CHILD LANGUAGE USE

They mix at school and at home, it suits them best.

Our kids use the mother's language together.

Japanese researcher, Masayo Yamamoto, Professor of Bilingualism at Kwansei Gakuin University, conducted several studies of Japanese-English child-to-child bilingual language use from a sociolinguistic perspective. The parents were usually following an OPOL strategy and lived in Japan, with one parent having a British or American nationality. In 1985 Masayo observed 24 pairs of children, and found that 19 of them chose Japanese as their 'main language of communication'. The other four either used English or mixed. She replicated the study in 1990 and found similar overall results: seven out of 13 sibling sets preferred Japanese (in this case four sibling sets used English, and two mixed both languages). The siblings who used English were usually attending an International school. Masayo conducted a larger study on 118 Japanese-English families, with 167 children, which formed the basis of her 2001 book *Language Use in Interlingual Families: A Japanese-English Sociolinguistic Study*. These data showed that around half the children used only Japanese and around half of the children mixed both languages. Only 5% of the children used English (the minority language) together. However, the majority (85%) of the children attended local Japanese schools, and played with Japanese-speaking children. Although many of the children had friends who spoke both languages. The chance to practice English for most children was limited to just one parent and one sibling. In the home, Masayo observed that when the Japanese parent spoke Japanese the children *always* replied in Japanese. Curiously, the child did not always reply in English with the English-language parent; he or she might reply in Japanese or a mix of both languages, which was accepted by the parent. This suggested that the country language had a strong influence on home language use and the English-speaking parents were more 'tolerant' of the children using Japanese in the home. The less practice they had using English, the less motivated they were to use that language with a sibling. Less practice meant less fluency and eventual passive use. As Masayo explained,

> In cases where all the children in the family have an equal command of two languages, they may choose a common language for several pragmatic reasons. It may be more convenient for them to choose the language used at school, if they go to the same school. They may want to use the societal language to include monolingual friends in their conversation, or they may choose the minority language for exclusionary purposes. If they are not fluent in a particular language, however, the chances are slim that they will use this language unless they are placed in situations where they must. (Yamamoto, 2001: 72)

I asked the 105 families, who completed the online survey, to say which language(s) their siblings used together. We have to rely on their personal assessment of the sibling language use, since it was not possible to verify exactly which language the children spoke together in private. However, I think most parents eavesdrop and have a good idea of the language their children use behind closed doors or when playing independently together. The information the parents gave allows us to see some patterns of inter-sibling language use within the families. One hundred and two parents reported on which language the siblings used together. In three families the siblings had not yet chosen a preferred language or spoke different languages. I asked the parents:

What language(s) does the child prefer to speak to his/her siblings in?

The data showed that the 74 sets of siblings in my survey had five different ways of communicating: using only the father's or mother's language, a mix of languages, the same language as their two parents spoke (these were children whose parents both spoke the same language but the family lived in a country or attended school where a different language was spoken) and a country and/or school language, which was *not* a parental language (Figure 3.1). Here are some examples of language use from the online survey families.

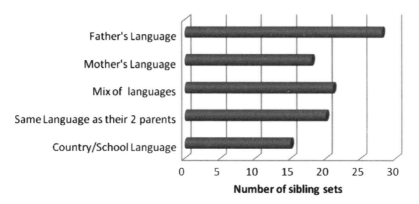

Figure 3.1 Sibling's preferred language

Father's Language as sibling's preferred language (28 sibling sets)

Family #95 lives in Mexico, which is the father's country. The mother is American. The grandmother and the nanny, who look after the children regularly, speak Mixteco (a Mexican dialect) to the children. Their four-year-old twin daughters attend a Spanish-speaking preschool and prefer to speak Spanish together. They speak Spanish to both parents, although the parents are trying to encourage more English use at home. The girls prefer to be read to in English, because the mother clarifies, 'We have more English books.'

Mother's Language as sibling's preferred language (18 sibling sets)

Family #72 is a German/English family living in England. The parents each speak their own language at home. The two young children, aged 5 and 3, speak German together. They both attend English-language schools and watch television and read books in either language. However, they have a German au-pair living with them, who encourages the children to speak German at home too.

Mixed Language Use (21 sibling sets)

> Family #11 is an English/Korean family living in Seoul. The mother is American. Their two boys attend Korean-language local schools. At home they mix Korean and English in their conversations, copying their parents who also mix both languages too. They also adjust their preferred language to the location, as the mother reports: 'In Korea, they speak more Korean together than in America. I notice that they have more English vocabulary'. The children have spent a lot of time in America. The brothers watch television in both languages, and the older one, who is seven, can read in both languages.

Same language as their parents (20 sibling sets)

> For example, Family #37 is a Danish family living in Belgium for the father's job. They have maintained a Danish-speaking home. The oldest child goes to an English-language school, and the younger one attends a Danish-language crèche. Together, the siblings always speak Danish and the parents are strict about language use in the home, expressly requesting that the language is only Danish. The family plans to return to Denmark in two years.

School or country language (15 sibling sets)

> Family #44, a Portuguese/German bilingual couple living in Israel, have two children aged 12 and 10 who prefer to communicate together in the country language, Hebrew. Both children attend school in Hebrew too. Hebrew is also the second language of both parents and has become the family's 'lingua franca'.

I had expected to see more mixing in the families, in line with Masayo Yamamoto's findings. The low number of mixed language use (21%) suggests that siblings prefer a more monolingual way of communicating together. Could this be related to the fact that they are enrolled in monolingual schools, which encourage exclusive use of one language? This area of language preference in children is often underestimated by researchers. Since children spend a large part of their day either at school or with school friends, it would probably have an effect on the language preferences one or more siblings unconsciously make at home.

THE SCHOOL LANGUAGE EFFECT

After the oldest one started school they quickly switched to using the 'school' language together and only used my language at home with me.

In studies on siblings observed by the parent-linguists and researchers the school language often becomes the majority or dominant language for children. Starting school is often a catalyst for a change in attitude and language use at home. Barbara Zuer-Pearson, author of *Raising a Bilingual Child* (2008), conducted a study with her colleague, Arlene McGee, on 110 junior high school students in Miami. They found that first-generation immigrant children switched to English within a very short time of arriving in the country. Barbara added that even children in dual-immersion schools, who were able to maintain their Spanish, still preferred to switch to English in the shared areas such as school halls, canteens and on the school bus.

Researcher Sarah Shin observed 12 bilingual Korean-American first graders in a school setting and interviewed 251 Korean parents of school-age children. In her book *Developing in Two Languages: Korean Children in America* (2005), Sarah highlighted the important factor of schooling. After the children entered the monolingual American schools their Korean language skills dropped. For first-born children, Korean-language use with their parents plummeted from 78.8% to 43.1%; Second-born children went from 66.3% to 26.8%, while the third-born children declined from 42.9% to 23.8%. Mixed language use and English increased in line with the decrease in Korean, with half the first-borns preferring to mix languages after they started school. Sarah concluded:

> The children, across birth-order categories, spoke more English (or Korean and English) and less Korean with their parents once they started school. However, even before entering school, fewer second-born children (66.3%) than first-born children (78.8%) spoke Korean with their parents, while even fewer third-born children (42%) did so. (Shin, 2005: 131)

The same scenario was seen in Una Cunningham-Andersson's English/Swedish household in Sweden, where once the youngest child joined the three older ones at a local school, the language of the siblings became Swedish. In a trilingual household, the school language can squeeze out parental languages. Charlotte Hoffmann remarked on her two trilingual German/Spanish/English children's change of language after the youngest child, Pascaul, started attending a local English-language school around age five. Charlotte understood that English was their most proficient language and the one they both spoke with 'the highest degree of grammatical accuracy.' She described the new situation,

> The children used to speak German to each other; however, now that Pascaul has been going to primary school for a year, he normally uses English as the language of play and explanation to his sister, and even to the parents. When asked to switch to German or Spanish he used to do so quite willingly, although he is becoming more reluctant now. It is clear that English is already his preferred language. (Hoffmann, 1985: 485)

A parent and researcher, Cathy Benson-Cohen, observed 39 language patterns of seven- to eight-year-old French/English bilingual children living in France. The parents reported that French usually became the dominant language between siblings once one or two children started nursery school. In an article from *The Bilingual Family*

Newsletter published in 2005, Cathy explained how French became more present at home,

> Once a child starts nursery, it appears that gradually more and more French is used to the English-speaking parents (who in all cases in this study is a competent French speaker). It is understandable that the child finds it easier to talk about events in French that happened in the French-speaking environment. However, once the child starts using French regularly to the English-speaking parent, they are less likely to push themselves in English. (Benson-Cohen, 2005: 5)

Fabiana, a case-study parent with four trilingual Italian/Chinese/English-speaking children, echoes the strong school-effect on sibling language use. In her family, the two eldest daughters began speaking Italian together (the mother's language) but soon changed to using English after they started attending an English-language school. Fabiana says,

> *Before starting school the girls were all speaking Italian between themselves. Our third child was already exposed to English through her sisters speaking English among themselves. Now all three prefer English.*
> Fabiana: Italian/Chinese/English trilingual family in Malaysia, mother of Martine (10), Natalia (9), Arianna (6) and Thomas (1)

Why does school have such a strong effect on language use? Dr Sarah Brewer, author of *A Child's World: An Unique Insight into How Children Think* (2001) says that children at primary school typically spend more than 40% of their day with their friends. Sarah describes the changing perspective of school-age children,

> Up to this point in their lives, children have tended to judge their own worth mostly according to the feedback they receive from their families and close friends. From now on, however, children's sense of self is increasingly based upon their relationships with their peers, as well as their performance in school and sport. Once children start spending more time with their peers, they have to follow new rules appropriate for these new social groups, and they start forming new impressions of their own identity as they re-evaluate themselves in the light of their peers' reactions and responses to them. (Brewer, 2001: 231)

Bilingual children who were keen to speak both languages in the tight family circle of preschool might be tempted to change their language use when they start school. This is especially pertinent if the chosen school is monolingual where bilingual children might think twice about speaking a language publicly that few people understand. The pressure is also increased by increased time away from home and after-school enrolment in activities in the local area, like sport or music. The risk is that the home or minority languages might fade away over time. From the children's point of view this is not necessarily a rejection of the minority language, more a pragmatic choice made by the children that since they spend so much time at school or with school friends. For parents who are able to make the decision about which school their children attend, they should carefully consider the language of school and activities and the possible effect it might have on their children's language use in the home.

Two case-study mothers, Alice and Martina, shared stories of growing up in bilingual families. Alice grew up trilingual; speaking German and Korean with her parents and attending an English-language International School in Korea. Alice and her brother, Oliver, began to speak English together, as she describes,

> *I grew up trilingual. We spoke German at home; Korean was the majority language and English we acquired later on in International School. As a five-year old I used to be fluent in Korean. We have tape recordings in which my older brother and I chatter and sing along in Korean. I remember speaking Korean with ease to my Korean grandparents and cousins. When I was in third grade elementary school, we returned to Korea (after spending time in Austria) and our parents sent us to an International School, where we acquired English. Even though we spoke German at home, my brother and I started to speak to each other in English, especially when we were together with friends or when we discussed our homework. I asked Oliver why we did this, and his response was "We just thought it was cool" – and I agree! Additionally, I would always turn to him, rather than my parents, for help with my essays, and we always chose to discuss in English, not German. Speaking English was easier, more logical for us in this context.* (Alice: German/Spanish/English in Austria (Lingua Franca), mother of Isabella (5) and Dominik (2))

Martina's parents sent her and her brother to an International School in Caracas. They preferred to mix Spanish and English (often referred in Hispanic communities as *Spanglish*). Here Martina recounts her childhood with two languages.

> *I was born in Caracas, Venezuela to Argentinean parents who spoke Spanish. My father learnt English as an adult by working in the US and my mom learnt English, "on the streets" as she says … meaning that she did not get an education in English. When we were born, my father worked for a multinational company and foreseeing that maybe we would end up moving to the US we got sent to Escuela Campo Alegre (an American school in Caracas). So we spoke Spanish at home and English at school. We traveled to the USA, twice while we were 12 and 14 yrs old, we went to a summer camp for a month in Georgia and another one in South Carolina. Since then, my brother and I have always spoken in English or Spanglish, together, and it's a special bond that came from learning English at school, more than just a language it was a way of life.* (Martina: Spanish/Italian/English trilingual family in Italy, mother of Alessia (8) and Gaia (6))

Was the school language a factor in the choice of a preferred language between siblings for the families who completed the online survey? Would siblings choose to use the school language together, or a parental minority language or a mix of two or more languages? To see if there was a pattern, I asked parents what language was used at school, and linked this information to the sibling's preferred language. One hundred and one families replied to this question, while four families had children who were too young to attend school. I asked the parents:

What is the language used in school and home between siblings?

Same school language and home language (47 families)
    Forty-seven sibling sets used the *same* language together at home and at school (Figure 3.2). The majority (40 sets) of these children used English at school and at home, and had one English-speaking parent. In general, these children were attending English-language monolingual schools (in America, Great Britain or International schools around the world).

Monolingual at school/mixed language at home (19 families)
    Nineteen families had siblings who attended monolingual schools. At school they used *one* language and at home they *mixed* two languages. This organization often functioned as an effective way to support a minority-language-at-home.

Family #26 is a French/English bilingual family living in England. All three children attend school in English and mostly speak English with their monolingual friends. At home, the siblings mix languages as their preferred way of communicating. As the French-speaking mother reports 'It can be French or English, depending on what activity they are doing. French is usually for books at home, or English for a television program they all watch'.

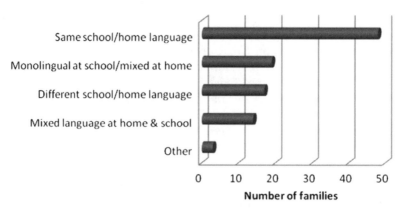

Figure 3.2 School/home language use

Different school language/home language (17 families)

Seventeen families had siblings who attended monolingual schools in *one* language. At home the siblings spoke *another* language together. This pattern was often seen in families who were maintaining a minority language in the home. Typically, the children were young (under six years) and had not yet started formal schooling. This pattern was also applicable to expatriate families who were temporarily living in another country for a few years and who were maintaining the parental language at home. Depending on the length of stay in the country and the school friendships built up, the majority language could stay an outside language, or over time, replace the parental language as the sibling's preferred language.

Family #87 is an English/Czech family living in Prague. The mother speaks English to her two young sons. The children attend local Czech schools. At home the boys speak English together. They both like to watch television in English and read English books.

Mixed language use at home and school (14 families)

Fourteen families used *mixed* language in *both* school and home. Ten sibling sets attended bilingual schools (usually with English as one of the languages). Four families lived in communities (Jordan and Wales) where mixed language use was common, and practiced by both adults and children.

Family #31 lives in Wales with bilingual Welsh/English parents, in a community supportive of bilingualism. The parents speak both languages fluently and mix. Their three children attend bilingual Welsh/English schools. All three children prefer to speak Welsh to their parents and Welsh together as their preferred language together, but switch easily into English depending on the topic. For television or reading, the siblings have no preference.

Apart from the 17 sets of siblings who specifically spoke a different language at home, there was a clear link of school-home language for the siblings. This would be expected since most parents choose a school with one parental language. However, the school language does seem to have a negative effect when it suffocates the minority language in the home. For half of the families the siblings chose to only speak the school language, giving the minority language very little chance to be practiced. The main reason for children using both languages at home appeared to be maintenance of one parental language (usually the mother's language) which is at risk of being overtaken by the majority or country language. In this respect, the children are sensitive to the potential loss of one language and are making efforts to avoid its passive use at home. This could be because the siblings have a particular bond through the minority language (shared experiences or memories) or because they appreciate the value of speaking the minority language to communicate with extended family or when visiting the country.

> The *school* language can be a strong factor in deciding the sibling's choice of preferred language. It is often an *older sibling* who inadvertently introduces the language of the school, or brings local friends home, and tips the language balance toward a school language.

MIXED LANGUAGE USE

> *Sometimes Child 1 will start a sentence in English and finish it in Spanish …*

> *My second son constantly mixes the two languages to the point he adds Hungarian tenses to English words. The first-born never did this.*

> *When they were little, they would germanise English words, for example, by adding "ge" in front of an English verb for the past tense (the toilet was "geflushed") or they would sometimes use German words in an English sentence (e.g., "it is donnering" – Donner = thunder).*

Barbara Zuer-Pearson, author of *Raising a Bilingual Child* (2008) observed a wide range of families in the United States and commented,

> In my experience, when children are left to their own devices, they almost always use the majority language (or code-switch heavily) with their siblings. (Zuer-Pearson, 2008: 151)

What is mixed language or code-switching? Mixing is when a child uses two languages together to form sentences and is a common occurrence in bilingual families. Mixing usually begins around age two, a time when the child begins speaking two languages. Research on young bilinguals and detailed transcriptions of children using both languages has led to mixing being accepted as a natural part of development and not a speech problem. At an early age mixing is usually a transitional stage while the two languages are acquired. There is some debate over the question of whether mixing is a sign that the child is not yet aware that he or she has two languages, or whether it is an early sign of the ability to switch languages to suit the person they are talking to. Mixed language use can cause worry initially, for some parents, as it appears that the child is having problems becoming bilingual or speaking either language well. Mixing is often referred to in academic terms as *codeswitching*. Parent-linguist Harriet Jisa describes codeswitching as,

> Code switching is a widespread phenomenon in bilingual speech communities and in conversations between bilingual individuals. Just as monolinguals may

switch registers, styles or voice during conversation, bilinguals may switch languages. (Jisa, 2000: 1364)

Much research has been done in this area, notably by Naomi Goodz (1989) and Elizabeth Lanza (1992), who studied bilingual children in their homes. Elizabeth Lanza's work in 1992 on a two-year-old bilingual girl Siri showed that she mixed languages with her Norwegian father, who accepted her mixing, but rarely mixed with her monolingual American mother. Elizabeth Lanza concluded that very young children, even at age two, are able to utilize mixing as a sophisticated way of talking to both parents. Naomi Goodz studied the effect of parents on mixing in four families. Goodz was particularly interested in the difference in parental attitudes toward mixed language. She found that although the parents claimed to follow a strict OPOL strategy at home they often mixed languages themselves, or accepted mixing with their children. This kind of mixing was often used to attract attention or discipline. Goodz concluded that,

> ... in bilingual families, parents will tend to choose words and linguistic structures that they are fairly sure the child will understand even if these words are drawn from the vocabulary of the other parent's language. (Goodz, 1989: 41)

Mixing also has a function as a sophisticated way of inter-family communication. In older children and adults mixing forms a social function as Colin Baker describes in his book *A Parents' and Teachers' Guide to Bilingualism* (3rd edn). Colin lists some major uses of codeswitching and comments on the reasons for why people codeswitch,

> To make a point, stress an argument, report something somebody else said more authentically, highlight warmth of friendship, and sometimes exclude people from a private conversation, code-switching isn't interference or mixing-up languages. It's a third subtle language that bilinguals use to clever effect. (Baker, 2007: 58–59)

In my survey, mixing was common in one out of three families. This parent in a German/Portuguese family makes the point that mixing is only done with other bilinguals,

- 30% of families had children who regularly mixed languages.
- 23 of the 105 sibling sets used mixed language use as their *preferred* way of communication.

They can sometimes use German words when speaking Portuguese and vice versa. This only happens in a bilingual setting.

In Family #13, a Danish family living in England, the children use a mix of Danish/English together. They both attend local primary schools locally. Their mother reports there are times when mixed language use is more common, observing:

They mix more often when they return from school in the afternoon. And more English words tend to be within their languages at the end of the school year. Since they are both bilingual they understand each other perfectly.

Mixing has a function in that it can form a social bond within the family with mixes that everyone understands. Some siblings or one sibling might use mixing as a language game, creating unique combinations designed to make other siblings laugh or as a private language together. Mixing is often heard when bilinguals are taped or videoed talking to each other privately, or in a community where both languages are regularly used. More structured mixing can be an accepted way of using both languages, often seen in families living in bilingual countries or in families who have chosen to follow a *mixed* strategy has been chosen (see Appendix 1 for more on the *mixed* strategy).

> *Mixed* language use is often a feature of early bilingual development. Later on it can bring siblings and family members together as a way of bonding socially.

SIBLINGS HELPING TO MAINTAIN A MINORITY LANGUAGE

My children speak my language fluently, and with ease, with me, but whether they will speak the minority-language with their brothers or sisters is quite another story.

It often seems, in theory, that as long as parents make the effort to provide enough minority language exposure and encouragement a child will become fluently bilingual. Parent-linguists Werner Leopold, George Saunders and Traute Taeschner all spoke the minority language to their children. The parents succeeded in having their children use the minority language fluently with them and concluded, rightly so, that their child was bilingual. This was true, to a certain point, but when the parents were not directly involved in a conversation the same children often preferred to use the language of the country/school together. Therefore we can say that the minority-language-speaking parents were successful in having children who spoke their language to *them*, but less chance persuading *all* their children to speak it together, regardless of careful efforts and planning. The Caldas children, for example, had approximately equal exposure to both languages, planned bilingual schooling and regular visits to Quebec, and still the siblings chose the majority language. This happens even when parents have the best intentions to speak their own language and have chosen a strategy, such as *OPOL* or *minority-language-at-home* to encourage maximum use of the minority language in the home. In real life, even the best bilingual parenting is not enough. With no or little inter-sibling language use, a minority language will become passive or underused over time, and the whole family could even slip into using the majority language together. It seems relevant that the minority language *has* to be used by the siblings too, at least in some way or form, ideally when the parents are not around or listening in. Since totally banning a country or school language or not allowing local friends in to play is not possible, parents may wonder how to keep the majority language at bay. How can we readdress the balance and encourage more minority language at home with two or more children? Leonore Arnberg discussed this problem in her book *Raising Children Bilingually: The Pre-School Years* (1987) and made the valid point,

> It is very difficult to solve this problem short of trying to generally increase the use of the minority language among the older children, for example, through spending time in the minority language country. More time can also be spent in family activities during which all family members speak the minority language together, or the minority-language-speaking parent may try to spend more time alone with the child. Parents may, of course, try to explain to older children the importance of their speaking the minority language to the child, but this has not been found to have a very long-lasting effect. (Arnberg, 1987: 120)

As Leonore says, family activities or language games could be a way to encourage older inter-sibling minority-language use. The three Saunders children often played games in German together (albeit mostly when their father was present) which gave their minority language a diversity it might not have when just used between parent and one child. George Saunders was able to tap into his children's love of jokes (often bilingual and playing with word meanings on both languages) to encourage more use of the minority language in a relaxed and informal way. Motivation and support from the other siblings might also have a role to play in keeping minority-language use alive, and allowing siblings to use it when parents are not present. Some parents enlisted the help of older siblings to help sustain a developing parental language. Charlotte Hoffmann expressly asked her three-year-old daughter, Christina, to play with her baby brother in German (the mother's language). As Charlotte recounts,

> In our case the older sibling contributed to her young brother's development of German **and** English: when Pascaul was born I asked Christina to speak to him in German so that he would hear this language from two different members of the family – a point which she fully understood even at that early age (she was 3 then). Until Pascaul started going to school full-time this agreement was adhered to. Even though her German was not perfect the fact that he heard German from another child who understood him, played with him in this language and shared his interests must, I feel, have contributed a great deal to his development of German. (Hoffmann, 1985: 492)

Although the intense German-language use between the children lasted only a few years, until both children started attending a local English-language school, it probably gave Pascaul a boost. Later on, Charlotte employed German-speaking au pairs to help encourage her children to use more German at home. There also appear to be some 'triggers' where children will automatically use the minority language together, without realizing it. In the Taeschner family the two girls, Guilia and Lisa, usually spoke Italian together. While recording discreet audio tapes in the background of the room where they played Traute noticed that even the presence of their mother in the room could lead to the children to switch languages (i.e. speaking

German to each other, not to her). There was no direct conversation or request from their mother to speak German, more an intuitive understanding that they should change languages in her presence. The girls would also switch to using German together to capture her attention, usually in sorting out a dispute over property. As Traute notes,

> On the few occasions when the girls spoke German to each other, there was usually a reason. Sometimes they wanted their mother to understand what they were saying. (Taeschner, 1983: 222)

How present was the minority language in the daily communication of the siblings in my survey? I asked the 105 surveyed families for data on their language use. Figure 3.3 shows language choices for 102 sibling sets (three sibling sets had not yet chosen a preferred language).

As the graph shows, almost two-thirds (63) of the sibling sets communicated in the language of one parent, which was also the *majority* language (i.e., the language also used in the country where they lived, and usually the language of school). These majority language-speaking siblings usually lived in monolingual countries, such as the United States and Britain. In these households a minority-language such as Finnish, Greek, Dutch, Slovak or Japanese was limited in practice and input. In such a family the country/school language risked becoming over-dominant and reducing opportunities for children to use the other parental language. When the children did speak the minority language it was only with one parent. This was made worse if the parent had few friends speaking that language around them or if the children felt uncomfortable speaking that language in public. These children certainly were bilingual, but the majority language had a clear dominance in their lives.

A mix of *majority/minority* was the norm for 19 of the sibling sets in the survey. This served a purpose in keeping the minority language use active. Seventeen sibling

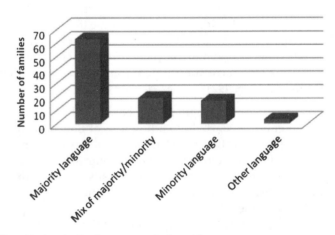

Figure 3.3 Minority/majority language choice at home

groups used the *minority* language together. Within this group nine sibling sets were using the mother's language compared to just one set, who spoke the father's language. However, there were seven families where *all* the family members spoke the minority language (either living as expatriates or practicing second-language-at-home or minority-language-at-home strategies). Three sibling sets were trilingual and used a *third* language, that was not parental, but a majority school and/or a country language.

Unfortunately, it seems that the majority language tends to crowd out the minority language over time. This could be linked to the cultural expectations of monolingual countries and schools. For example, in the United Kingdom and the United States, being bilingual is still unusual and a risky strategy for older children, and teenagers wanting to fit in to their respective peer groups. The minority language can possibly be maintained through joint family activities or immersion in countries or activities where *only* the minority language is used. For example, the Caldas family made frequent trips to Quebec, where the children felt comfortable speaking French together. Children who are able to integrate both majority and minority languages into their conversations may well come off the best in the long run, as they establish a relationship based on both languages and can create their own unique dual language culture. The real issue is whether children feel comfortable speaking the minority language in their world, or with children of their age. If this is the case, families with minority-language-speaking parents can benefit from having their children speaking their language within the family. Not only does it give the parent someone to communicate with on a daily basis, it also strengthens the language exposure for the whole family. Unfortunately, many siblings naturally gravitate to majority language use over time. Siblings cannot be forced or coerced into using a particular language with a sibling, especially if it restricts their communication.

> In some families, minority language use could be *maintained* and strengthened through inter-sibling use.

SUMMARY

In this chapter we have seen that siblings in bilingual families need a language for their private communication. This preferred language is usually, but not always, a parental language. Survey families and case studies report that the sibling's language is usually the one used in school or in the country where the family lives. The society the children are brought up in can be a strong force to be reckoned with. We must bear in mind the importance of time spent at school and school friends in the choice of preferred language; it is to be expected that this will weigh on the children's final choice of language. This is most profound in a monolingual country or culture. Many sibling sets choose to mix or switch from language to language, thereby pleasing both parents and creating their own unique mix along the way. Children in trilingual families, with parents speaking two different languages and living in another country, appear to prefer the neutral choice of the country or school language.

The role of the minority language and the siblings is a complex one that needs more investigation. Published case studies acknowledge the success of a child to communicate in both languages with a parent, but this is only one side of the story because the sibling preferred language choice needs to be taken into account too. The relevance of the role of the minority language in the whole family should not be underestimated. If siblings willingly use the minority language *together*, there is more chance that the language will stay 'alive', rather than fade away. Certainly minority-speaking parents facilitate and control language use when children are young but can the siblings maintain it as the family grows? Typically, families with young children (under age five) were more likely to be using the minority language together. As they move into their teenage years it can become harder for parents to impose their language preferences on their children. Consequently, in Chapter 4 we will take a closer look at the factor of age difference and the number of children in the family.

Further reading on sibling relationships

Arnberg, L. (1987) *Raising Children Bilingually: The Pre-School Years*. Clevedon: Multilingual Matters.

Baker, C. (2007) *A Parents' and Teachers' Guide to Bilingualism* (3rd edn). Clevedon: Multilingual Matters.

Benson-Cohen, C. (2005) Oral competence and OPOL: Factors affecting success. *The Bilingual Family Newsletter* 22 (4), 4–5.

Caldas, S.J. (2006) *Raising Bilingual-Biliterate Children in Monolingual Cultures*. Clevedon: Multilingual Matters.

Cunningham-Andersson, U. and Andersson, S. (1999/2004) *Growing Up with Two Languages: A Practical Guide*. London: Routledge.

Goodz, N.S. (1989) Parental language mixing in bilingual families. *Infant Mental Health Journal* 10, 25–44.

Hoffmann, C. (1985) Language acquisition in two trilingual children. *The Journal of Multilingual and Multicultural Development* 6 (6), 479–495.

Jisa, H. (2000) Language mixing in the weaker language. *The Journal of Pragmatics* 32 (1), 363–386.

Lanza, E. (1997a) *Language Mixing in Infant Bilingualism: A Sociolinguistic Perspective*. Oxford: Oxford University Press.

Shin, S.J. (2005) *Developing in Two Languages: Korean Children in America*. Clevedon: Multilingual Matters.

Taeschner, T. (1983) *The Sun is Feminine: A Study on Language Acquisition in Childhood*. Berlin: Springer-Verlag.

Yamamoto, M. (2001) *Language Use in Interlingual Families: A Japanese-English Sociolinguistic Study*. Clevedon: Multilingual Matters.

Zuer-Pearson, B. (2008) *Raising a Bilingual Child*. New York: Living Language/Random House.

Note: You can read more about the families of Fabiana, Alice and Martina in *Family Profiles* at the end of the book.

Chapter 4

Age Difference, Family Size and Language Orders

We saw in the previous chapter how siblings choose a *preferred* language and set the stage for family language use. This chapter discusses the factor of the age difference between children and the size of a family, alongside related issues of siblings having varying loyalties to family languages due to age differences, and older siblings taking on a teaching role in the family. We begin with a look at the difference between siblings who are close in age (two years or less apart), and those siblings who have a wider age gap (three or more years). How does this age difference affect the inter-sibling language use? Parents often observe that their older siblings 'teach' younger ones. Do older siblings naturally take the role of teachers? Could that benefit bilingual families and help the parents maintain minority languages in the home?

We also investigate how the number of children in a family might affect family language use. Do three or more children create a dynamic language environment, or does having a large number of children dilute the chances of the children being bilingual? The chapter ends with a discussion on families who have children speaking different first or second languages in a bilingual family. Why do some siblings have different 'first' languages or language orders? Could a difference in age lead to children having different language dominances? Throughout this chapter there are examples from the case studies on bilingual and multilingual families in Chapter 1, alongside comments from participants in the online survey on age difference, family size and siblings as teachers.

CLOSE-IN-AGE SIBLINGS

Ella, 4, and Benjamin, 2, have spent two years together at home with their French-speaking mother. They live in Belgium and their father is British. Ella is Benjamin's playmate, role-model and entertainment when their mother is busy. They watch television together and often choose the same programs or DVDs. They frequently go to visit other French families for an afternoon *gouter* or snack. Their mother, Anabel, reads to them together at bedtime, usually in French. Ella chooses the first book and Benjamin the second one. They share a room and toys, most importantly, a box full of costumes that they both love to play with. In September, Ella will start going to the nearby international English curriculum preschool. Ella tells her brother that she will teach him to read and write too, and she will make him a class-room in their room. Anabel worries that when Ella begins school she will want to do things without her brother and speak more English at home than before.

Close-in-age siblings can be loosely defined as children born with two or less years between them. Children that have such a close age gap often have similar lifestyles, like Ella and Benjamin. Children born with less than 28 months between them have very little recollection of life without a sibling. On a practical level they may share a room, attend the same playgroups or preschools, do the same activities or sports and share friends. Their cultural background may be similar, watching the same television programs together or reading the same books. Psychologists Stephen Bank and Michael Kahn (*The Sibling Bond*, 1997) discuss the way that close-in-age siblings share 'parallel lives', saying,

> They share much with each other, but the sharing is two-edge: the children can develop a common language about the same world, each knowing what the other is talking about. Yet by virtue of their closeness in age they may also collide and struggle with one another more frequently. (Bank & Kahn, 1997: 27)

In terms of language, close-in-age siblings may share a 'secret' language together. Close-in-age siblings can often understand the other one almost instinctively. The siblings may invent composite words from each language, add grammatical endings or adapt expressions from one language to the other. This secret language might be used between siblings at home or in public as a private code, which outsiders do not understand. Little research has been initiated on the issue of whether the age gap can have an effect or not on language use. In a small-scale study in 1978, Keith Nelson and John D. Bonvillian studied siblings and the rate they acquired languages. They found that 'short-lag' second-born children (i.e. a younger sibling with a gap of less than 24 months) were better in tests of syntax and concept development. The short-lag children outstripped both first-borns and later-born siblings with a wider age gap. Nelson and Bonvillian concluded that the second-born children profited from their family position, interacting and imitating their older siblings. Often just listening in to an older sibling can increase conversational abilities. Barton and Tomasello (1994) studied the language interaction of 19 sets of a mother, child and a young sibling. The older children were aged from three to five years old, with siblings aged from 19 to 24 months. Their results confirmed that when a mother was talking with her two children there was a beneficial effect. Interestingly, the younger one was able to 'eavesdrop' or listen in, and pick up useful knowledge on vocabulary, conversational skills and turn taking. Barton and Tomasello explain,

> … the mother-sibling-infant triadic context not only provided many opportunities and some practice at joining into ongoing conversations between other persons (something that is never possible in a dyadic context), but fostered increased and extended conversational interaction as well. (Barton & Tomasello, 1994: 129)

Several of the parent-linguists in Chapter 1 had close-in-age siblings. Often the parent intended to only transcribe the older child's language development, but was unable to ignore the presence of the chatty second-born child. For example, Traute Taeschner German/Italian girls, Lisa and Guilia, were just 13 months apart. In fact, Traute Taeschner's book was primarily a study on Lisa, but since Lisa mainly talked to her sister, Guilia, at home Traute was obliged to include their shared dialogue in the book. The study was enriched by the sister's chatting and Traute was also able to compare the girls at certain ages. Likewise, another parent-linguist, Harriet Jisa, had two English/French daughters close in age, Odessa and Tiffany, who had 15 months difference. In a study on their language use while staying with their grandparents in America Harriet described how the girls became immersed in English over the summer holidays. Tiffany was just beginning to speak English and learnt the rules of code-switching through her older sister's example. The girls switched and mixed English with French together, with the comforting knowledge that even if the monolinguals around them did not understand them, at least their sister could. A two-year gap is common; George Saunder's two sons had a two-year gap, as did two of Tracey Tokuhama-Espinosa's three children and the children in the Caldas family. There were two years between Madalena Cruz-Ferreira's three children and in the Cunningham-Andersson family two of the four children were close in age. In all of the bilingual parent-researcher families, the close age gap was seen as beneficial because the younger ones arrived in a family where not only one parent was speaking a certain language, but also a brother or a sister too.

The bilingual families I interviewed agreed that supporting a minority language at home was easier with a close-in-age set of siblings who shared books, films and, most importantly, used the minority language together. The early shared cultural references and memories of language in action could help reinforce future language development, especially if the siblings spoke the minority language, or a mix of both languages, to each other. Several parents thought that being a second-born child with a sibling just a few years older was an advantage in terms of language stimulation. Although it could be confusing at times, as Claudia observed,

Milo and Zeno are 2 years and 2 months apart and I can see Zeno being immensely stimulated by his older brother; at 18 months he has a richer vocabulary than Milo had at the same age. The second born has one more individual to look up to (the older sibling), who speaks all of the languages involved at once. This definitely has an impact. There are three adults who speak each a different language (mum, dad, nanny/teacher), and there's a little brother who uses all three. It must be puzzling somehow.

Claudia: Italian/ Flemish/ French/ English multilingual family in France, mother of Milo (4) and Zeno (2)

We see that young bilingual siblings who are close in age may not understand the distinctions of different languages, but are clearly aware that their older brother or sister speaks two, or more, languages. Within families following strict language strategies (like *OPOL* or *minority-language-at-home*), where each parent only speaks one language, the older sibling is likely to be following a different strategy. Each parent strictly speaks only one language. But the older brother or sister speaks *two* languages on a daily basis. How does the younger one comprehend this situation? Evidence from case studies suggest that the younger siblings appear to find it perfectly natural that their older sibling is following a different strategy, and we often see a similar pattern of language development in the early years.

> Close-in-age siblings can share similar lives, activities, cultural backgrounds and early *language patterns*.

WIDER AGE GAP BETWEEN SIBLINGS

> Phoebe, 7, and Nicolas, 12, were born in Italy. When Nicolas was four years old, the family came to live in England. Pheobe was born one year later. Nicolas had a lot of trouble adjusting to his new English-language school in the beginning, but once he made friends he spoke English quickly. Nicolas joined the local football team in Essex and practices several times a week. When Phoebe started primary school two years ago her brother was in his last year and she hardly saw him. Now he is at the local secondary school, which specializes in languages, and he is doing very well learning French and Spanish. Nicolas still speaks Italian with his parents, but rarely outside the home. Pheobe has her own group of friends and does hip-hop dancing and swimming after school. She mostly speaks English, with some mixed language use when the family is together. The children watch television together and enjoy helping their mother prepare Italian Nights, when they cook regional Italian food and invite their friends to eat with them.

A child three or more years older than a sibling will most likely have different language patterns, as we see with Phoebe and Nicolas. Siblings with a wide age gap of six or more years can behave as an only child or a first born. Even with a gap of just three to four years there can be a difference in daily activities and environments, for example, if the older one attends preschool or kindergarten and the baby stays at home with the mother or caregiver. On a positive note, a wider age gap can lead to a second-born child having more one-to-one time with a parent. A parent has potentially more time to chat, read, sing or play with the little one to encourage verbal skills. Linguistic interactions between a mother and her child have been widely studied. However, there is very little about mothers and two children.

A mother's way of communicating with a young child through simplified and direct speech, using special words to amuse the baby, is often referred to as *motherese*. Would a sibling copy the same *mothersese* when talking to a younger sibling? Michael Tomasello and Sara Mannle (1985) recorded the conversations of 10 sets of mothers, three to five-year-old firstborn children and their 12–18-month-old siblings. The older siblings in their study did, in most cases, replicate *motherese* in their conversations with younger siblings, especially when a parent was around. But this was not always the case. In fact, Tomasello and Mannle (1994) found that frequently an older sibling would not always respond to the younger one. In detailed transcripts they found that 83% of the words or short sentences spoken by the infant were simply ignored by the older sibling. This compared to 21% of ignored utterances when the infant talked to the mother. On top of this the older siblings frequently changed topic or used language that was too sophisticated for the infant. When Tomasello, Barton and Mannle retested their findings, with infants aged 22–28 months, the same effect was replicated. The researchers concluded,

> Together, the results of these studies of sibling–infant conversational interaction indicate that although preschool-age children do use some features of motherese speech, they are not as adept as mothers at making pragmatic adjustments for younger children. (Tomasello *et al.*, 1994: 123)

In spite of having a rather uncommunicative older sibling, the younger sibling was actually challenged to keep up with the conversation. Barton and Tomasello thought that the sibling's inter-language use prepared children for the real world of peer friendships and school. Having a mother who listens to everything you say and asks you lots of questions was useful in the early years, but not always so helpful in a preschool or primary school environment. A child who is only accustomed to their mother's focused and adapted speech might struggle to communicate with a group of strangers at school. The older sibling effectively showed an insight to the real world, where conversations have to be initiated and maintained to form friendships. Tomasello and Mannle argued that later-born children might grow up to have better conversational skills,

The directiveness of siblings and their nonresponsiveness in conversations may contribute to the tendency of some later-borns to employ expressive styles of language acquisition. (Tomasello & Mannle, 1985: 911)

One common trait with a wider age gap is that older children can have a tendency to 'talk down' to younger ones. Judith Rich Harris (*No Two Alike Human: Nature and Human Individuality*, 2006) noted the way siblings can 'talk-down' to their younger brothers or sisters, or any child younger than them,

> … studies have shown that children as young as four 'talk down' to still younger children, just the way parents do, in an effort to make their speech understand-able to the younger child. The four-year-olds use simpler, shorter sentences when conversing with two-year-olds than with children of their own age. They do it whether or not the younger child is their siblings and whether or not their par-ents are present. They do it even if they don't have a younger sibling. (Harris, 2006: 97)

What about the parents-researchers with children who had a three or more year age gap? Did a wider gap make a difference? The widest age gap was in the Leopold family where the two girls, Hildegard and Karla, had six years between them. This age difference meant that Hildegard's German was well established when Karla was born. Nevertheless, Karla was described as having 'passive' bilingualism, after many years hearing her father and sister conversing in German. Theoretically, Karla should have benefited from her fluent German-speaking sister. Perhaps because her sister was so prodigious at languages, or perhaps because her father spent so much time with her sister, Karla never spoke both languages as well as her sister. We do not know much about the language use between the sisters, but over time Leopold reported that Hildegard spoke less and less German as she moved into adolescence and became closer to her American peer group. Karla's passive German finally became active when she went to Germany as a teenager. Fantini's children, Mario and Carla, had a four-year gap between them and there were three years between Christina and Pascual in the trilingual Hoffmann family.

In these families the older sibling was often in a different phase of language development when the younger one arrived. The older siblings had more contact with the outside world of school and local friends and were, by nature of the age gap, more skilled at languages than the younger. In the Saunders family, the third child, Katrina, was born five years after her two brothers. Katrina benefited from her father and older brothers speaking German around her. According to her father, she learnt to read and write in German, before starting at her local English-language school. With the encouragement of her two bilingual brothers and father at home, Katrina was encouraged to speak the minority language at home. Katrina was soon able to join in family games (generally conducted in German) and follow conversa-tions at home.

I asked some of the case-study families what they thought about age gap and bilingualism.

We found that with a three-year gap, our older son was already very proficient in the language and could help his little brother. Our youngest then also had the advantage of being able to listen to his older brother and me speaking together.
Christina: English/German in Germany (OPOL), mother of Tom (15) and John (12)

When combined with birth order and gender, a large age gap can sometimes make the oldest child a 'decision maker' in the family. This was the case in Josie's family, with three boys who have three or four years between them. Asked if she thought that an age gap mattered in a bilingual family, Josie commented that sometimes the older children teach language the parents would prefer them *not* to have learned (e.g. swearwords or playground slang).

Our boys are relatively far apart in age (4 years and 3 months between the first two and 3 years and 8 months between the younger two). The big age gap matters here in the sense that the oldest child could determine if one language should be the dominant or only language spoken between the boys and which one. It may well be that Tobias stopped speaking English to me following his older brothers lead, although I can't be sure about that as we were living in Germany again by the time he made the switch. In the first year back in Germany, Tobias still spoke English and stopped just before he started school at age 6. The older sibling certainly helps in language growth in our family, although the words the younger ones learn are not what I would usually want to hear used so regularly.
Josie: Chinese/German/English trilingual family living in Germany, mother of Niklas (12), Tobias (8) and Lukas (4)

We see that the older sibling could show a 'good' model of how to use language appropriately. Children with a wider gap may communicate differently, with less playing and more teaching. Even if an older sibling may not pay much attention to a younger one or interact directly with him or her, they can show how to switch topic or language.

A *wider* age gap may lead to older siblings teaching or influencing younger ones. An older sibling who is talking fluently shows an alternative to parental language models.

SIBLINGS AS TEACHERS

Our first child is often 'teaching' our second and third children by modeling 'Say x ....', and then correcting them afterwards.

Are older siblings natural teachers, for better or for worse? Psychologists, Judy Dunn and Carol Kendrick (*Siblings: Love, Envy & Understanding*, 1982) observed older children clearly adjusting their speech while talking to their baby or toddler sibling,

In practice all the children, even those as young as 2½ years, changed their speech dramatically when talking to their baby siblings. Their speech to the baby consisted of much shorter utterances than their speech to their mothers, and it contained a high frequency of repetitions and of attention-getting utterances. (Dunn & Kendrick, 1982: 124)

This can be seen in the way first-borns simplify their speech for the little one, copy a parent's way of talking or refine their choice of vocabulary. Dunn and Kendrick also observed that the older child's language was often adapted to 'prohibit, dissuade, or restrain the baby', along the lines of 'No, Don't do that!' or 'Stop! Put it down!' This may seem negative, but in context, bossy language use was probably needed because the baby/toddler brother or sister was at an age when he or she needed to be controlled or disciplined. The older sibling was echoing the parent's voice and language patterns too. Judy Dunn (*Sisters and Brothers: The Developing Child*, 1985) commented,

> The more 'parent-like' behaviors of teaching and care-giving are more frequently shown by older children in families where there is large age gap. (Dunn, 1985: 80)

Charmian Kenner (*Becoming Biliterate: Young Children Learning Different Writing Systems*, 2004) studied six bilingual children in London, observing the dual language worlds of children whose parents spoke a minority language at home and who attended English-language schools. The children she studied often attended Saturday schools or 'complementary' schools for extra minority language input. Charmian noted the complexity of living with two languages and how older siblings could play a role in guiding younger children how to use each language appropriately. The older siblings often employed the same teaching techniques as used in the school environment. One family had a particularly strong sibling support. Six-year-old Ming was being brought up with English from the community and two Chinese languages, Hakka and Cantonese, at home. Ming had five siblings ranging in age from 12- to 24-years old. Charmian observed the following sibling interactions,

> Ming's older siblings, particularly his twelve-year-old brother, helped him with his homework from Chinese Saturday school. On Thursday or Friday evenings Ming practiced writing the characters. He knew his brother could translate and would ask him the meaning of Chinese words in English. (Kenner, 2004: 7)

Charmian also noted how Ming would read his school library books to his brothers and sisters and watch how they used English/Chinese dictionaries for their secondary school or college homework. His sisters helped him practice writing his name and to do informal activities at home, such as making a Christmas card. The effort made by the siblings to support biliteracy was very positive and helped Ming to go further with his emerging bilingualism through the older sibling's encouragement and experiences. Had the parents in my study found an older sibling took on a teaching role? I asked parents if they agreed with the statement:

An older child will usually help teach a younger child to speak a language

This question provoked a positive 'yes'. The majority of parents, two-thirds of the 105 families, agreed with the statement and thought that an older child would usually help a younger one learn languages (Figure 4.1). There were 12 families who

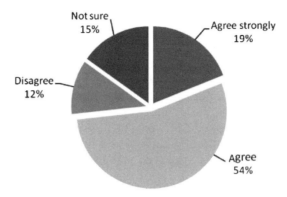

Figure 4.1 An older child will usually help teach a younger child to speak a language

disagreed with the statement and 15 parents who were not sure. Here are some comments from the parents I surveyed on their children's teaching techniques:

When my second child was learning to speak, using Portuguese in Israel, her older brother would correct her and provide the Hebrew equivalent, saying 'This is what WE say' …

Our oldest child often helps his brother and corrects his pronunciation, either in Portuguese or English. He does so very emphatically and has his younger brother repeat a word until he can say it right …

Andrea, mother of a teenager and two young children, thought a wide age gap was more conductive to sibling teaching. Andrea's two daughters, Lena and Melanie, both took on teaching roles.

In our case, the age gap works as an advantage since our older child (Melanie for both the little ones, and Lena for Finlay) was/is at an age where she can perceive herself as a model and teacher.
Andrea: English/German in Germany (L2 at H), mother of Melanie (15), Lena (6) and Finlay (3)

Canadian mother, Christina, found that the first-born was a strong role model in her family too. Tom, now a teenager, used English with his younger brother, supporting and encouraging the use of the minority language at home in a German-speaking environment.

The first child may get more intensive language input since the parents don't have to divide up their attention between two or more children, But other children have the advantage of being able to learn from their siblings. We found that already having one bilingual child helped to reinforce our goal. Our older son acted as a 'helper' to teach his younger brother English.
Christina: English/German in Germany (OPOL), mother of Tom (15) and John (12)

Like monolingual siblings, several parents commented that their children had picked up language patterns directly from siblings, citing slang, swearwords or accents that the parents did not use themselves. Some parents said that their older sibling helped the younger ones with tricky grammar, pronunciation or vocabulary. How far should parents go in allowing older siblings to 'teach' a younger one? Parents from the case studies also reported that some older siblings took on the task of correcting younger ones emerging language use. In other families an older one would try to tell the parents, or other adults, what the little one was trying to say. This is a common scenario, seen in both monolingual and bilingual families. However, in a bilingual family, one language could be dangerously under-used and become passive. Around a third (34 out of 101) of the parents said that one of their children (usually the first child) 'talked' for another. Here are some comments from parents via the online survey on an older sibling 'talking' for a younger one,

My son interprets what he thinks his sister (age just over two years) is saying ...

My son speaks for his sister. He has a firm belief she can't understand French because she doesn't speak it. But she understands French 100% ...

Our second child did not speak until age 3 due to the first one speaking for her.

Kendall King and Alison Mackay in their book *The Bilingual Edge: Why, When and How to Teach your Child a Second Language* (2007) discuss the issue of younger children needing extra help. Kendall and Alison recommend that parents are vigilant in not letting older children speak on behalf of younger ones, as they say,

If older siblings take on the role of translators for their younger brothers or sisters, encourage them to let the younger children speak for themselves. But also encourage them in their role as language tutor. (King & Mackay, 2007: 82)

Translating or talking on behalf of a younger sibling can help in some situations, like when a child is shy and is reluctant to use one language or lacks enough vocabulary to reply to someone. But it could lead to a sibling who is over-reliant on the other sibling's linguistic prowess. A big sister can take her maternal role very seriously. This is done with the best of intentions, but it can result in a brother relying heavily on his sister to talk for him or vice versa. This scenario was seen in the Tokuhama-Espinosa home with Natalie, their first-born daughter, and their second-born son, Gabriel. In this diary excerpt Natalie is three and a half, and Gabriel is 13 months. After a family move from Ecuador to America, Gabriel was not talking yet and Tracey was concerned:

It seems to me that he spends all of his brain power on learning to master gross motor skills like walking, throwing, bouncing, and banging, and little if any energy on speaking. He is so different to Natalie .... Is this because he is a boy? A second child? A second child in a bilingual family that had just changed language strategies on him? Yes on all counts, his pediatrician at Harvard said to us last week. Add to those three factors a fourth, she said, which was an overly helpful sister who translated his every need into a clear verbal request. (Tokuhama-Espinosa, 2001: 169)

By the time Gabriel was three, he had found his voice and learnt to 'interrupt' his sister's constant narrative by saying 'Nati, it's my turn, my turn' Interestingly, a few years later, when a third child was born, Gabriel found himself with a new role as teacher to his younger brother, Mateo. Having an older sibling who is keen to tutor a younger one can be a positive factor. Younger siblings can benefit from listening in to conversations between parents and siblings. A teaching role, through role playing, can exist between siblings. However, children should not be pressurized to be a teacher at home. An overly helpful child can sometimes unintentionally stifle or talk for a younger one, a situation that can lead to a child being frustrated and missing practice in speaking one or both languages. All in all, parents should not leave language learning solely in the hands of a sibling.

Siblings can *teach* younger ones and show an example of how to use each language in context. Some older sisters (or brothers) may *talk* or *translate* for a younger sibling but younger siblings need practice and should be encouraged to talk more.

FAMILIES WITH THREE OR MORE CHILDREN

In the survey, two-child families were prevalent, which is typical in European and North American families. However, 16 families had three children and seven had four children. In three families there were two sets of siblings living in the same house, with parents who had remarried. There also were five sets of twins (of which one set also had four other siblings).

- 77 families had two children
- 16 had three children
- Seven had four children
- Three families had stepchildren
- Five sets of twins

In a two-child family, the children only have each other to talk to. In families with three or more children would there be more opportunity for language interaction? Would the children support a minority language at home? Four of the families discussed in Chapter 1 had three or more children: Saunders, Tokuhama-Espinosa, Cruz-Ferreira and Cunningham-Andersson. In the Saunders family, Frank and Thomas were close in age (two years between them). This was beneficial to their sister Katrina, who arrived in a family where bilingual language use was established and three people already spoke German. This was echoed in the Tokuhama-Espinosa trilingual family where the third-born child arrived in a stable established language environment and the siblings used all of the languages at home. In Madalena Cruz-Ferreira's Portuguese/Swedish/English trilingual family the three siblings kept the minority languages of Swedish and Portuguese active, as did the four children in the Cunningham-Andersson family.

Their reports were generally positive in nature and praised the complicity and shared cultural background and minority language use in the home.

However, for the 23 survey families with three or more children, it was a different story. Looking at the families with three or four children it appeared that the country language, or the majority language, became the first language of the siblings and the one they used together. The minority languages appeared to fade away over time. For example, Family #46, a Finnish mother and an American father, living in America. Their four children, a boy born in 1992, and three girls, born in 1994, 1998 and 2002, all speak English first and Finnish second. The mother reports that her two oldest children have an 'intermediate' knowledge of Finnish, while the third and fourth children have a 'beginner' level. However, their mother described Child 3 as only 'having a few sentences in Finnish' and Child 4 as having 'just a couple of words in Finnish'. The mother reports,

> *When the two oldest started school and realized that no one else spoke Finnish and Mom knew perfectly well English, they decided they were done using Finnish ('no one speaks that language Mom'). I spoke with the two youngest Finnish when they were first born and I was home by myself with them, but as soon as the family walked in from school, it was back to English. The two youngest just weren't exposed to Finnish enough and never really used Finnish.*

This was replicated in the other survey families with large families. The third or fourth child typically spoke only the language of the country where the family lived, despite having one or two parents and two siblings who are bilingual. In the families where the children did use both languages it was because they attended schools in the minority language. Minority-language use was strong while the children were young (children aged 5 and under) but when they started school the situation changed. With three or more children enrolled in a local majority-language school the minority language appeared to decline over time. What did the case-study families that I interviewed think about the number of children in a family and its effect on bilingualism? Seven out of the 22 families had three or four children. Gerry, a Canadian mother of four English/Spanish children, thinks that the more children the better in terms of language use. Gerry notes that parents can profit from having time with a younger child, while the older ones are at school, as she notes,

> *The saying, 'the more the merrier' comes to mind. With so many people chatting in so many languages at once, it has its effect on the whole picture! I have personally seen three different languages being used at any one time, in numerous ongoing conversations in our home. I think that the number of children does affect the way parents communicate and use their languages with their children and when gaps occur in birth ages (like when a few years pass and another baby is born) it is easier to spend more time with the later born if the previous (older) child is already more independent or at school, for example, leaving more time for mom or dad to communicate and be with the new baby.*

Gerry: English/Spanish in Canada (OPOL), mother of four children (aged 13, 11, 7 and 5)

However, other parents felt that a large family decreased the chances of the minority language being used, in line with the findings of the survey families. Theresa, mother of three English/Spanish girls living in Spain thought that language skills would be improved by having two or more siblings, but not necessarily in the minority language.

> *With two or more children, I think there is a tendency for them to use the language of the country they live in when talking to each other. Language growth in general may be stimulated by having siblings, since there are more opportunities for communication, but for second language acquisition it may be a hindrance.*
> Theresa: English/Spanish in Spain (OPOL), mother of Carmen (13), Rocio (11) and Violeta (9)

Fabiana has three daughters and one son. In their Italian/Chinese/English trilingual family in Malaysia, the parents are encouraging the girls to speak the minority language of Italian (the mother's language) to their little brother, alongside some Chinese (one of the father's languages). Fabiana plans to involve the older siblings in teaching the younger one some Italian and Chinese but is concerned that the minority languages lack support, as she explains:

> *I personally fear that the more the number of kids in a bilingual family the lesser chances the minority language has to survive. I speak Italian to the children and the kids speak Italian to me. My husband speaks English to the girls and Mandarin to the baby. The girls go to an international school where they speak English and study Bahasa Malaysia as second language. They also have been taking Mandarin classes for years and they are just learning to converse in this language. Among themselves they use English. I also asked the girls to use Italian with their little brother rather than English. They sometimes enthusiastically, sometimes reluctantly try to do so. They understand and feel the importance of it.*
> Fabiana: Italian/Chinese/English trilingual family in Malaysia, mother of Martine (10), Natalia (9), Arianna (6) and Thomas (1)

Tammy is the mother of four daughters close in age. The American parents, of Hispanic descent, speak Spanish to their four daughters. They follow a minority-language approach at home and two of their daughters attend an International school with a Spanish section. Nevertheless, the girls prefer to speak in English and the family is struggling to keep Spanish active.

> *We now sprinkle more English into the home whereas when we just had Isabel we were more exclusive to Spanish. Our second daughter, Elena, did not speak until age three due to Isabel speaking for her, Elena then mixed both languages until she was about age 4, and now mostly speaks just English. Although we both still speak to all of them in Spanish, because they do not respond back, their Spanish skills have deteriorated. Since they know we are more fluent in English, they do not want to speak to us in Spanish.*
> Tammy: English/Spanish in the United Kingdom (mL@H), mother of Isabel (8), Elena (6), Monica (3) and Nora (1)

A large family can give more language variety and models of language use. There is more diversity in the language use and more opportunity for younger siblings to copy or imitate older ones. Having an established bilingual strategy in the house could encourage and support minority language use as research and case-study families found. Nevertheless, there is the question of whether a minority-language would be 'lost' over time, as more siblings join the family, and whether the minority language would become passive in a larger family, as the survey families reported. This is difficult to prove, with such small numbers of families in my study, and with each family having unique combinations of languages, siblings and particular circumstances. However, we can say that in the families with three or more children, certain 'group' identity exists, with one inter-sibling language becoming dominant, and the effect could be stronger than in a two-child family. With three or more children refusing to speak a minority language, it is perhaps harder for parents to reverse the situation than for one or two children. In such a situation the parents cannot really do much, except perhaps change the language of school, or move to live in a country using the minority language, where the children would have more exposure and chance to use that language.

SIBLINGS WITH DIFFERENT LANGUAGE ORDERS

Do all siblings speak the same languages? Do they all have the same dominant language? Parents in bilingual families might find that one of their children has more fluency and confidence in speaking in one language, while other siblings may have differing language patterns. In the online survey I asked the parents to list their child's languages, in order of the child's preference, as their first language, second language and third and fourth language (if applicable). The first language is the language which is most dominant in the child's overall language use. It is often the mother's language too, but not always. In school-age children (aged five and above) the child's most dominant language is usually the school language. Here are the results of the language preference question:

What languages do your children speak, in order of preference?

In 64 families all the children spoke the same languages with the same order, that is first, second or third (Figure 4.2). This would be expected in line with research done on bilingual families. In 18 families, one or more siblings were not yet talking fluently and parents could not judge which language was their strongest. Curiously, one in five families (23) had siblings where one child's first language was different to a sibling's first language. It was often a reversed pair of languages. Child 1 spoke Language A as their first language and Language B as their second language, while Child 2 spoke Language B as their first language and Language A as their second language.

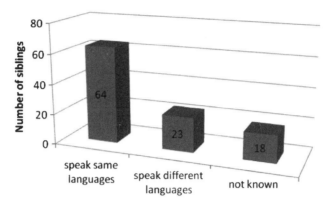

Figure 4.2 Children speaking the same or different languages

	Child 1	*Child 2*
First Language	Language A	Language B
Second Language	Language B	Language A

Why did these 23 families have children speaking different languages? In many cases, this was due to the age gap between siblings. A typical scenario was a family with parents speaking two languages and living in the father's country. One sibling speaks more of the mother's language while the other child speaks more of the father's language. Both siblings are bilingual, just with more of a leaning toward one parental language. The younger sibling was immersed in the home environment and spending much of the day with his or her mother. The older sibling was already at school, the language of the community or their father, and that language had become their strongest or 'first' language over time. The same pattern was seen in families with three or four children.

For example, Family #7 lives in Kiev, Ukraine. The mother is American and the father French. They have a Russian-speaking nanny. Their two children were born in 2000 and 2004. Child 1 speaks (in order) French, English and Russian, while Child 2 speaks English, French and Russian. Child 1 is currently attending a French-language international school, while the younger one is at home with her mother and the nanny.

Family #26 is trilingual. The mother is French, the father Turkish and they live in England. They have three children born in 1998, 2001 and 2005. The two oldest children are boys and speak (in order) English, French and Turkish. The third child, a girl, has French as her first and strongest language. All three attend English-language school (or daycare) but the third child, who is just 2½ years old, only goes in the mornings and still has more affinity with the mother's language.

In nearly all of these families, the youngest child was in the two to five years age range. This meant that in a few years the situation could change rapidly as the younger sibling joined older ones at primary school. Starting full or part-time preschool at age three or four years can be a potential trigger for a change in language dominance. In the English/Swedish household of the Cunningham-Andersson family, there was a move from dominance in the mother's language (English) to the language of the country and the father (Swedish) at around age three. The mother, Una, noticed that this coincided with the four children starting school, as she says,

> The children were all English-dominant until they started pre-school at around age 3 years of age. Now they are all very clearly Swedish-dominant. (Cunningham-Andersson, 1999/2004: 32)

There were some families in my sample who had moved homes between births of successive children from one parent's country to another, or to a country where another language was spoken. Often this meant a change of language too. A Korean-English family had spent five years in the father's country (America) and then moved to Korea. Their first-born son was proficient in English which was his dominant language. Korean was difficult for him to practice outside the immediate family. His sister was born just before they left to live in Korea with family. She became dominant in Korean, and was looked after by her grandparents in the early years, but she had the reverse problem of lacking opportunities to speak English. Over time, the language order stabilized and the children evened out when they both attended the same English-language school, with Korean as the community language.

There were some families where older siblings were particularly attached to one language, through a different school language, cultural activities, sports or friends. One sibling might not share the same interests and be more attached to the 'other' language. Becoming a teenager could have an effect too. This was seen in the Caldas family, with two preadolescence and one adolescent child. In the fifth grade, the older son, John, moved to an English-language High School, while his twin sisters continued their French-language immersion schooling exactly two years behind him. John's dominant language became English and his cultural attachment to that language increased while the girls' first language was French, as they stayed closely affiliated to their mother's Quebec roots.

These language order differences linked to age difference are often short-term or temporary, and as a younger sibling moves up and into preschool, primary school or secondary school siblings can align their dominant and minority language preferences. In other families, one sibling can remain closely aligned to one language, while another feels more comfortable using the other language.

Even siblings living in the same home, with the parents speaking the same languages, may have very different *language orders*, depending on their personal experiences of languages in their lives.

SUMMARY

The age of each sibling, the age difference between them and the size of the family can affect bilingualism, albeit in subtle and complex ways. Whether or not siblings benefit from being close in age or from having a wider age gap is varied. In both respects, the language interaction between siblings can be beneficial. Close-in-age children who have similar cultural backgrounds can support shared language learning in the future. Wider-age gap sets of children have the potential to teach and become a linguistic role model for younger ones. A minority language can be activated by having older siblings speaking it to younger ones. Likewise, an older sibling can prefer to *not* speak a minority language and that sibling can influence other children. Shared sibling interests, and time spent together as a family appear to be important in terms of increasing and maintaining minority language use. Parents can possibly increase language use too, simply by having conversations with two or more children. A younger sibling can still gain from having a sibling as an in-house model of bilingualism in action even if the older sibling can potentially ignore, 'talk down' or talk for them. The role of older siblings as translators and tutors should be carefully monitored by the parents, otherwise younger ones may lack practice and become too dependent on a sibling for communication.

Family sizes can affect bilingualism in that the more children there are the more chance that the minority language may be under-used. However, with more children there is more chance for children to listen in and acquire language from their siblings, giving a variety of speech models. Siblings may, at certain times in their lives, find themselves speaking different languages. Due to age gaps or different language dominance through schooling or language preference, there may be sibling variation or division. These reverse language orders, in many cases, realign with time or changing circumstances, such as when a younger sibling joins an older one at school. In Chapter 5, we take a look at the factor of gender and how boys and girls, or brothers and sisters, approach language differently.

Further reading on age gap and family size

Bank, S.P. and Kahn, M.D. (1997) *The Sibling Bond*. New York: Basic Books.

Barton, M.E. and Tomasella, M. (1994) The rest of the family: The role of fathers and siblings in early language development. In C. Gallaway and B.J. Richards (eds) *Input and Interaction in Language Acquisition*. Cambridge: Cambridge University Press.

Cunningham-Andersson, U. and Andersson, S. (1999/2004) *Growing up with Two Languages: A Practical Guide*. London: Routledge.

Dunn, J. (1985) *Sisters and Brothers: The Developing Child*. MA: Harvard University Press.

Dunn, J. and Kendrick, C. (1982) *Siblings: Love, Envy & Understanding*. MA: Harvard University Press.

Gregory, E. (2001) Sisters and brothers as language and literacy teachers: Synergy between siblings. *The Journal of Early Childhood Literacy* 1 (3), 301–322.

Harris, J.R. (2006) *No Two Alike Human: Nature and Human Individuality*. New York: W.W. Norton & Co.

King, K. and Mackay, A. (2007) *The Bilingual Edge: Why, When and How to Teach Your Child a Second Language.* New York: Collins.

Nelson, K.E. and Bonvillian, J.D. (1978) Early language development: Conceptual growth and related processes between 2 and 4½ years of age. In K.E. Nelson (ed.) *Children's Language* (Vol. 1). New York: Gardner.

Tokuhama-Espinosa, T. (2001) *Raising Multilingual Children: Foreign Language Acquisition and Children.* Westport, CT: Bergin & Garvey.

Tomasello, M. and Mannle, S. (1985) Pragmatics of sibling speech to one-year-olds. *Child Development* 56 (4), 911–17.

Family size

http://www.census.gov/population/www/cen2000/briefs.html. Accessed 10.3.10

http://europa.eu/rapid/pressReleasesAction.do?reference=MEMO/05/96&format=HTML &aged=0&language=EN&guiLanguage=en. Accessed 10.3.10

On WWW at http://www.pregnantpause.org/numbers/fertility.htm. Accessed 10.3.10

'Fertility Rates (Children per Family) World Statistics' (2001)

Note: You can read more about the families of Andrea, Claudia, Christina, Josie, Gerry, Theresa, Fabiana and Tammy in *Family Profiles* at the end of the book.

Chapter 5
Gender and Language

This chapter looks at the link between language and siblings. Young children often acquire stereotypical ideas about boys and girls, and prefer to play with children of the same gender. Generally, girls begin speaking earlier than boys and appear to have more interest in communicating through language, while boys are more interested in motor skills. However, there are many individual variations of this gender-specific behavior and not all children follow this pattern. The gender divide is often noticed in the early learning patterns of boys and girls, especially in educational terms. Are girls more disposed to speaking or learning second languages? Could this gender difference affect the children's developing dual language skills and their interest in foreign languages?

In terms of bilingual families there are some interesting issues. Young girls who speak earlier can be judged as 'bilingual at an early age', and there can be some unfair comparison with boys. This can affect parents trying to maintain bilingualism and concerned that they are doing something wrong. Some languages have specific male / female forms of communication. For example, in an OPOL family a girl could imitate the language patterns of her father, or a boy copy his mother. How do families with only one parent speaking a language balance gender-specific language practice? Throughout this chapter we also consider some of diary data from the bilingual families that were introduced in Chapter 1. These families will be discussed in this chapter in relation to gender, along with comments from the bilingual and multilingual families that I interviewed via the online survey and case studies.

THE GENDER DIVIDE

In the 1960s, behavioral and developmental psychologists working with young children showed that children are aware of the differences between males and females from around age two onward (see the early work done by Kohlberg (1966), Maccoby (1966) and Slaby and Frey (1975) for more on this area). A two- or three-year-old child can accurately identify a person as a girl, boy, mother or father. However, they may not be sure of the stability of the situation yet, therefore they can think that a boy can become a girl, or vice versa, simply by putting on dressing-up clothes or changing a hairstyle. Preschool children may not be sure if they will stay a boy or a girl either. By age six or seven children are more aware of the gender difference and know that boys will grow up to be men and girls become women, regardless of the differences in appearance. But the gender difference creates a split. In a playground or preschool environment we often see children divided into two distinct groups; the boys running around the playground playing games involving physical activity, and the girls gathered together in small groups around the benches or sidelines. Dr Sarah Brewer (*A Child's World: An Unique Insight into How Children Think*, 2001) interviewed and observed children at school, and gave an accurate description of primary school age children's behavior:

> Girls tend to play more quietly in smaller groups, or stand around chatting. They typically develop one or two close 'best' friends with whom they have equal status and will go out of their way to avoid conflict. Girls bond with other girls through talking, sharing secrets and forming close emotional ties. (Brewer, 2001: 124–125)

In contrast, boys tend to hang around in larger groups and indulge in rough and tumble horseplay. Boys are also more likely to resolve conflicts through physical means and settle differences with their fists. Male friendships are more likely to be based on shared activities and interests, such as sport, rather than being underpinned by sharing emotional confidences. Gender norms can be so strong in a group context that some children who do not behave in a typically girly or boyish way can be excluded or teased. Even when parents and teachers try to treat boys and girls equally, and give them the same toys and choice of activities, children continue to stereotype gender. Robin Banerjee, a lecturer in Psychology at the University of Sussex, argues that children have strong beliefs, saying in a 2005 online article on Gender Development:

> In fact, the beliefs of children in these early years of childhood can be much more strongly stereotyped than the beliefs of most adults … Moreover, the children act on these stereotypes. Especially as young children begin to play more and more with peers of their own sex, we begin to see striking differences in the ways that boys and girls play. (Banerjee, 2005: 1)

Gender is often portrayed in stereotypical images in books, films or television programs for children, with boys kicking a football around or running about shouting at each other, while the girls talk to their dolls or pretend to be princesses. These stereotypes could serve a purpose in simplifying a child's world and creating unwritten rules about social behavior within a group. As they get older, children become more aware of the flexibility and individual nature of gender too, for example, accepting that a girl can play with cars or that boys can dance. Gender is closely linked to the expectations and assumptions of the society the child is brought up in. Each culture or society has its own specific rules on what is acceptable behavior for boys and girls, which might reinforce certain masculine or feminine qualities. Parents also model appropriate behavior and reinforce certain ways of dressing, speaking or behaving according to the child's gender.

At school, some teachers may treat boys and girls differently and sometimes have different expectations of the work they should do. Typically, girls can be more drawn toward language, drawing, writing or reading projects. Boys may be more interested in making things or doing sports or scientific projects. Nevertheless, these generalizations do not apply to all children, or teachers, and there are many girls who enjoy science and many boys who read enthusiastically.

Many children go through a period where they follow stereotypical behavior patterns based on their *gender*. This often coincides with children growing up and learning how to fit into the social world of peer groups outside of the home.

GIRLS, BOYS AND LANGUAGE

In terms of language development there can be a slight difference in the way that boys and girls communicate. Parents often report that girls begin talking slightly earlier than boys. Why do the girls talk earlier? Family therapist Steve Biddulph in his book (*Raising Boys*, 1997), specifically for parents and their sons, reported on the differences between male and female brain wiring and the increased levels of testosterone in boys. Testosterone is often linked to increased physical activity, aggressiveness or 'boyish' behavior. Testosterone also effectively blocks the brain from using its left side temporarily at certain ages, especially when testosterone levels run high around age four and at puberty. Male brain development is more right-sided in the beginning, with a focus on problem solving, mathematics and spatial awareness. Since language development is situated in the left side, boys can take a little longer to 'grow' into using their language-orientated left side. This might help explain why young boys lag behind girls with early language development and sometimes have problems settling down to formal schooling at age four or five. Biddulph emphasizes that the hormone imbalance does not affect all children in the same way and the child's home environment and school is important too. Parents who encourage verbal interactions, reading and literacy at home with their sons can help them 'catch up' with their female counterparts.

The female brain has a larger *corpus callosum*, a band of nerve cells connecting the left and right sides of the brain. This helps the two sides to communicate faster and allows girls to use both cerebral hemispheres simultaneously. A team of researchers (see Harasty, 1997) found that in females, the two parts of the brain which are closely linked to language learning are 20–30% larger than in male brains. Further research is still needed to establish whether the brain is like this at birth or if it is stimulated by language practice. By using fMRi (functional magnetic resonance imaging) scans, researchers have found that male brains develop more slowly and that female brains utilize both sides, left and right, and make more connections between the two sides. Interestingly, bilingual brains utilize both sides of the brain too, and so bilingual boys may well have the same early advantage that girls have.

In the field of Neuroscience and Linguistics, several studies have been conducted to see if there is a gender effect. One study on 55 young first-born and second-born sibling pairs (Bornstein *et al.*, 2004) observed that some children can have a linguistic advantage related to their gender. The researchers found that first-born girls outperformed the boys on all the vocabulary tests, and second-born girls scored better on all the tests put together. A similar study conducted by three researchers from Northwestern University and the University of Haifa, (Burman *et al.*, 2008) used fMRi to measure brain activity in 31 boys and 31 girls (aged 9–15 years) while they performed spelling and writing tasks. These tasks were visual (pictures) and auditory (sounds). The study highlighted the fact that girl's brains worked harder, since the areas of the brain used for language were activated quicker. The girls processed information in an 'abstract' way, while the boys had a more 'sensory' approach. The girls were simply more effective at understanding the problem and using more parts of their brain appropriately. Girls were better at remembering word lists or 'mental lexicons', but young girls made mistakes with overgeneralization, or applying the same rule to everything. For example, saying 'I *holded* the bunny', instead of 'I held the bunny'. On the other side, the boys excelled at the grammatical details of language, they preferred lining up grammatical rules to make up each sentence, rather than using the same formula each time. This could lead to the girls talking faster (even if they make more mistakes) while boys need a little more time to 'build' their language.

Anecdotal evidence from parents points to the fact that girls might excel linguistically because mothers talk more to their daughters than their sons. A meta-analysis of data on parents talking to their children (Leaper *et al.*, 1998) concluded that mothers talked more to their daughters than their sons, and used more 'supportive' speech than fathers. Therefore, it would make sense that girls acquire more vocabulary at an earlier age, especially if they have the benefit of a mother who talks a lot to them. Girls might have higher levels of comprehension too, because they pay more attention to the details of a conversation or the underlying messages. Parents might expect more of their daughter's language skills and consequently encourage their daughters to talk more at home. Psychologist Gisela Preuschoff (*Raising Girls*, 2004) thinks that daughters do have an advantage, saying,

> Parents speak more often to their female babies, which certainly could explain why girls seem to listen more attentively. As girls maintain eye contact longer

than boys, they 'demand' that their parents devote more time to them, smile at them, talk to them. (Preuschoff, 2004: 6)

Girls might have an emotional advantage too. Janet Kuebli (1995) and two colleagues listened to children aged three, five and six recounting past events (such as a trip to a park or a holiday). They found no initial differences with the younger children. But the five- and six-year-old girls were much more tuned into what the authors describe as 'emotionally-based' vocabulary or being able to talk about abstract notions such as sadness, happiness or feelings. The girls were able to get their messages across in a very specific and meaningful way, and had a wider variety of emotional or expressive vocabulary, compared to the boys.

If girls talk more than boys at an earlier age it could be simply because they have more practice through the games they choose to play too. The girls may have acquired the art of conversation through role playing and listening to each other in their smaller groups at school. This awareness of the usefulness of language might pay off at school because they are more articulate and able to answer questions and participate in discussions.

> Comparing boys with girls suggests that *girls* do have a different way of approaching language learning in the early years, but *boys* catch up over time.

EARLY-SPEAKING BILINGUAL GIRLS

Looking at the diary records from the parent-researchers and linguists in Chapter 1, who have observed family bilingual development and anecdotal evidence from families we can see some common issues relating to the gender of the child and their language use. When boys in bilingual families do not speak 'early', the parents can feel they are doing something wrong or following the wrong language strategy. Girls, on the other hand, prove that the parents are on the right track. In many families, the early years of establishing bilingualism are crucial in deciding whether they continue or not to bring up their children with two languages. Colin Baker (*A Parents' and Teachers' Guide to Bilingualism*, 2007) discussed the question of whether girls and boys differ in their progress toward bilingualism and biliteracy. He noted that girls tend to develop their verbal skills slightly faster than boys, but affirmed,

> There is no reason to believe that girls are better equipped to become bilinguals than boys. There is no reason why girls should be treated differently from boys (or vice versa) with regard to childhood development of bilingualism. (Baker, 2007: 55)

A two or three-year-old girl who is talking well in both languages is a very positive incentive for parents to continue and encourage her language use. Beginning to speak is a developmental milestone and parents understandably see their child's first words as 'proof' that they are doing the right thing. Anecdotal evidence from bilingual families and comments from families that I have interviewed for this book suggest that when a boy takes longer to speak one or both languages, questions are asked by the parents, family and friends. Take this example from a bilingual chatroom discussion:

> *Our 2-year and eight-month old son is not talking yet and seems more interested in building a castle than talking! Should we worry or just wait a while?*

A late-talking boy or a boy who has immature language skills may be referred to a doctor or speech specialist, who may recommend 'dropping' one language for a short time. Family and friends might remark that the choice of bilingual family language strategy is not right and suggest monolingualism as the answer to the language delay. The parents may well decide to abandon bilingualism or change their language strategy. In most cases the boy simply needs more time and bilingualism will usually emerge after a delay of 6–18 months.

Girls who start speaking early might 'prove' that bilingualism is working in their family.
Boys who start speaking late might worry parents that bilingualism is not working for their family.

FOREIGN LANGUAGES AND GENDER

Gender appears to be a factor in older children's attitudes toward learning second or foreign languages at school. In secondary school or high school teenagers can have very stereotypical ideas about language learning, which can affect their performance. The issue of gender in children studying Modern Languages at secondary schools has been a topic of research for several academics in the field of education. In national tests performed on children in England and Wales studying languages (usually French or German) up to GCSE level, there was a wide gender gap, with girls scoring well and boys underperforming. A team of researchers (Warrington *et al.*, 2000) concluded after a three-year study of a school in East Anglia, UK, that the problem was the issue of peer pressure and social image. They concluded that it was more acceptable for girls to work hard and still be part of the 'in-crowd', but for boys it was harder to be 'cool'. The boys risked being teased or bullied if they studied languages. According to a study by Beatrice Davies (2004) secondary school age boys have little motivation or interest in studying languages. They began with negative attitudes toward learning a foreign language in Year 7, and three years later still had little or no interest in the subject. Colin Baker (*A Parents' and Teachers' Guide to Bilingualism*, 2007) reports on the tendency in Wales for bilingual English/Welsh adolescents to abandon one language, saying,

In Wales, for example, there is evidence to show that boys tend to develop less favorable attitudes to the minority language compared with girls. Girls tend to retain their bilingualism and boys veer slightly more to English monolingualism in the teens and twenties. This partly reflects the behavior that gives status and peer approval, as well as mass media influences, and continuing parental and 'heritage culture' influence. (Baker, 2007: 55)

Another team of researchers (Williams *et al.*, 2002) interviewed 228 pupils in a school in South-West England. They discovered that the boys were more motivated to study German than French. It appeared that French was seen as being 'the Language of Love and Stuff' and not 'cool' for boys. The researchers noted that in many cases the teachers and parents reinforced such stereotypes. Language learning was a 'girl' thing in the eyes of the streetwise teenagers. However, the research on gender and adolescents at school is not conclusive and is often generalized, not allowing for the individual differences boys and girls can have. Each child has a different perspective on gender, and their individual experiences at school and home with boys and girls will affect them too.

Although these results were recorded on monolingual children, there can be a crossover with bilingual families. Girls may be keener to learn a second or third language, at home or at school. Families might find older sons keen to abandon a minority home language in favor of a school or community language. In the Caldas family their adolescent son, John, dropped French in high school due to peer pressure. In a monolingual environment, being bilingual is low priority for teenage boys. Boys may be reluctant to use a language if it affects their peer standing or leads to teasing from new friends. Families with older children who want to introduce another family language, or move to live in another country where a different language is spoken, might need to bear the gender issue in mind.

> Girls can appear more motivated in *learning languages* in general, when compared directly to boys. Social peer pressure can play a role with older children or adolescents and boys may be temporarily less inclined to *study* languages.

THE GIRL MYTH

What did the parents in my study think about gender? I asked them if they thought that girls had an advantage of linguistic ability, or is it just a myth? Are girls really better at learning languages than the boys? In my survey, there were 121 boys and 118 girls, who were more or less equally balanced for the first, second and third children, with slightly less females in each group (except for fourth children). I asked the parents to agree or disagree with the statement:

A girl will usually be more successful at becoming bilingual than a boy.

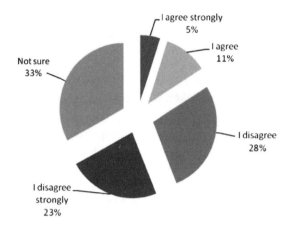

Figure 5.1 *A girl will usually be more successful at becoming bilingual than a boy*

	Boys	Girls
Child 1	55	52
Child 2	54	51
Child 3	11	10
Child 4	1	5
Total	121	118

Of the 105 parents who replied to this question the majority did *not* think being a girl was an advantage for becoming bilingual (Figure 5.1). Only 18 families (16%) agreed with the statement, while half families (51%) disagreed with the idea that having a daughter would boost bilingualism. A third (33%) of the families said that they did not know. Due to the limited nature of the online survey, is it not possible to know why they were not sure. I asked the case-study families if they thought that gender had any effect on their children's language use. There were five families with only daughters, five families with only sons, and 12 families with mixed boy/girl sibling sets. What did they think about the gender issue? About a third of the case-study families said they did not know, roughly the same number as the online survey parents. Some parents with only girls or boys were reluctant to comment on the gender issue, saying they lacked experience. Several families said that other factors were more important such as personality, age gap or how the siblings got on together. Here are some of their comments.

Gerry, Christina, Lilian and Claudia, all mothers of two or three boys, thought the girl issue was a myth. These mothers reported their boys, regardless of their gender, have all matured into excellent language speakers. They also noted that their boys started speaking early and had good language proficiency in relation to their age.

> *My sons, especially one, are very talented in languages. Girls are expected to be quiet and well behaved or studious, while it is acceptable for boys to focus on sports. Naturally the girls will have more varied experiences with learning and studying while the boys may have less, and vice versa. I believe that gender roles (thus*

expectations) are shaped strongly by the societies and cultural environments in which we live.
Gerry: English/Spanish in Canada (OPOL), mother of three sons and one daughter (aged 13, 11, 7 and 5)

Judging from our experiences with our boys, who started talking quite early and are very proficient at both languages, I'd say it is a myth.
Christina: English/German in Germany (OPOL), mother of Tom (15) and John (12)

I'd say it's a myth because my boys have both had excellent language development.
Lilian: English/Portuguese in the United States (mL@H), mother of Kelvin (5) and Linton (3)

I have two boys and they both developed linguistically flawlessly, without delay and without any problem. They began speaking at 14 months. At age three years and eight months Milo was fluent in Italian, French and Dutch, and shows a lot of interest for the English he has heard passively until now.
Claudia: Italian/Flemish/French/English multilingual family in France, mother of Milo (4) and Zeno (2)

Girls are better at languages!

There were some parents who thought that girls did have a linguistic advantage over boys. Jenifer, Toni and Nadya thought that their daughters did have some superiority in language terms. One mother, Josie, mother of three boys, thought that having a girl in the family might have changed things for them, in terms of increased vocabulary use.

I have seen in my family that my girl is more verbal. She was an earlier talker and got her grammar correct more quickly than my boy. I don't know if this is individual or a gender difference, however.
Jenifer: Japanese/English in the United States (L2 at H), mother of Lachlan (9), Kiki (5) and Case Kaye (1)

It seems true – all the little girls I know are so much more verbal!
Toni: Catalan/German/English trilingual family in the United Kingdom, father of Laia (4) and Elies (2)

Yes, I think that girls are better at languages, both in speaking skills and reading books.
Nadya: German/English in the United Kingdom (OPOL), mother of Elicia (5) and Charlotte (3)

Having only boys means I can't say so much on this topic. I do share the belief, though, that girls are, in general, better language-wise than boys. A girl in the family may well have increased the vocabulary of our boys.
Josie: Chinese/German/English trilingual family in Germany, mother of Niklas (12), Tobias (8) and Lukas (4)

Our son is the verbal one ...

There were also some parents who had expected their daughter to be the chatty child in the family and found, to their surprise, that their son was actually as good as, or in some cases, better than her. This is what Odile, Alice and Vicky said about their children.

> *I always thought girls would be better at {languages} but I'm in a position where it's actually my boy who's doing better, so I don't know now.*
> Odile: French/English in Malaysia (OPOL), mother of Amy (7), Luca (5) and Elliot (1)

> *In my family, it seems to be my son who is picking up languages with greater ease than my daughter. As a consequence I would say gender doesn't really matter.*
> Alice: German/Spanish/English in Austria (Lingua Franca) mother of Isabella (5) and Dominik (2)

> *I used to think that girls were better with language. But my younger son has, in the last couple of years, sped past his (non-biological) older sister in vocabulary, sophistication etc. in both languages.*
> Vicky: English/French in the United States (L2 at H), mother of Annis (10) and William (9)

Girls might speak like daddy or boys might speak like mummy ...

In some languages, there is a difference between male and female verbal language use. This can mean that men and women can use a slightly different grammar, accent or pronunciation. For example, Japanese is one language where the gender difference is defined.

Deborah Tannon is a sociologist who has researched male and female speech, saying that women use more 'rapport' and men 'report'. Female language can be more polite, include more rhetorical questions to find out about a person, and 'minimal responses', such as saying 'mmm' or 'yeah' in conversation. Male language can be more direct, with questions asked for a reason and less turn taking. In some cultures, certain slang words or expressions are associated with men or woman, and when used inappropriately they can sound wrong. Sometimes a young child inadvertently copies the speech patterns of an adult of the opposite sex. We might hear a little girl 'talking like a man', or vice versa, a young boy talking in a rather female manner. This is usually temporary, and can be amusing at the time. With enough examples of male and female speech around them children quickly pick up the subtle differences and use appropriate language use. However, in some bilingual families there is only one parent to give an example of language use.

A case-study mother, Lisa, found that her Israeli-speaking husband could not illustrate the female way of speaking Hebrew. She noticed that her daughters lacked some Hebrew language skills when they moved back to Israel after living in America, where her husband was the only speaker of Hebrew:

> *One thing we didn't realize when using the OPOL strategy is that our daughters were missing a large part of the language. In Hebrew, verbs don't only have person and number, they also have gender. So a man speaking to one or two girls leaves out many combinations. Female to two females. Female to male. Male to male. They were also hearing only parent to child dialogue – not peer-to-peer conversation.* Lisa: English/Hebrew in Isreal (mL@H), mother of Rachel (14) and Sarah (14)

Madalena Cruz-Ferreira is the mother of three Portuguese/Swedish/English trilingual teenagers. Madalena (personal correspondence, 2007) recounts how her two young daughters initially followed the norms of their father's 'male-Swedish,' while her son spoke Portuguese in a rather feminine way.

> Our girls started speaking male-Swedish like daddy and the boy spoke female-Portuguese like mummy! The issue was solved as soon as they all made friends with peers, including same-sex peers, who spoke these languages.

Una Cunningham-Andersson had a similar experience to Madalena with one of her four English/Swedish children. Una reports in her book *Growing Up With Two Languages: A Practical Guide* (1999/2004):

> The boy's use of their mother's language (English) may lack a masculine input, sounding rather sissified. Conversely, the girls' Swedish, with no mother's touch to moderate the father's speech, may have a tomboyish tone, such as Elisabeth (2;5): 'Nu ska vi käka' ('Grub's up!' – Literally 'Now we are going to eat', where kaka is a slang word for eat) which is quite inappropriate for a 2-year-old girl. (Cunningham-Andersson, 1999/2004: 54)

Una also commented on how children can learn a language or culture 'unevenly' from one parent. For example, a child can learn cooking vocabulary only from a mother in one language, and talking about football in the other language with their father. The children consequently lack the respective words in the other parental language. The problem of 'sounding wrong', or only knowing words from one parent, is easily remedied with more input or exposure from other speakers of the language. However, it is something to bear in mind if you are the only speaker of a language in the family.

A wide *variety* of language models are needed for young children, ideally with both male and female speakers.

SUMMARY

Gender appears to be a relatively weak factor, in terms of its effect on language use. There may be some early advantage for girls, who create more opportunities to converse with their parents or other adults, increasing their vocabulary and language skills. However, the bilingual families in my study were simply not convinced that girls are 'better' at languages. From the evidence in the case studies and from my survey families the bilingual boys seemed to be doing just as well as the girls, and many of them were speaking both languages from an early age. Whether this is because they use both sides of their brain when processing two languages or because their parents encourage their early language development is hard to say. More neurological and linguistic testing is certainly needed in this area.

Parents of boys who are not speaking both languages at an early age should not worry. Parents should not abandon language strategies because their son is not talking in one, or both, languages at an early age. Boys usually catch up in linguistic terms over the period of middle childhood or primary school. However, keeping boys interested in language once they reach adolescence is another challenge and may depend on the attitudes of the boy's peer group. Negative attitudes to one language from boys can set off a rapid and public disowning of a parental or minority language.

A wide range of language models is needed for young children to see the way language is used in both masculine and feminine ways, especially in those languages which have specific masculine or feminine grammars, accents or gestures. If gender can affect language use, would being the first, second or last child in a family make a difference? In Chapter 6, we take a look at birth order and how a child's place in the family can affect language use.

Further reading on gender

Baker, C. (2007) *A Parents' and Teachers' Guide to Bilingualism* (3rd edn). Clevedon: Multilingual Matters.

Banerjee, R. (2005) Gender development. On WWW at http://www.open2.net/healtheducation/family_childdevelopment/2005/gender_development.html. Accessed 29.4.08.

Biddulph, S. (1997) *Raising Boys*. London: Thorsons.

Bornstein, M.H., Leach, D.B. and Haynes, O.M. (2004) Vocabulary competence in first- and second-born siblings of the same chronological age. *Journal of Child Language* 31 (4), 855–73.

Brewer, S. (2001) *A Child's World: An Unique Insight into How Children Think*. London: Headline Books.

Burman, D.D., Bitan, T. and Booth, J.R. (2008) Sex differences in neural processing of language among children. *Neuropsychologia* 46 (5), 1349–1362. See also: Northwestern University (2008) Boys' and girls' brains are different: Gender differences in language appear biological. *Science Daily*. On WWW at <http://www.sciencedaily.com/releases/2008/03/080303120346.htm>. Retrieved 13.10.08.

Cunningham-Andersson, U. and Andersson, S. (1999/2004) *Growing Up with Two Languages: A Practical Guide*. London: Routledge.

Davies, B. (2004) The gender gap in modern languages: A comparison of attitude and performance in year 7 and year 10. *Language Learning Journal* 29 (1), 53–58.

Gender differences in spoken Japanese. On WWW at http://en.wikipedia.org/wiki/Gender_differences_in_spoken_Japanese.

Georgetown University Medical Center. (2006) Study of language use in children suggests sex influences how brain processes words. *Science Daily* 28 November 2006. On WWW at <http://www.sciencedaily.com/releases/2006/11/061127210527.htm> Retrieved 13.10.08.

Kuebli, J., Butler, S. and Fivush, R. (1995) Mother–child talk about past emotions: Relations of maternal language and child gender over time. *Cognition and Emotion* 9 (2/3), 265–283.

Kohlberg, L. (1966) A cognitive-developmental analysis of children's sex role concepts and attitudes. In E. Maccoby (ed.) *The Development of Sex Differences*. London: Tavistock.

Leaper, C., Anderson, K.J. and Sanders, P. (1998) Moderators of gender effects on parents' talk to their children: A meta-analysis. *Developmental Psychology* 34 (1), 3–27.

Loulidi, R. (1990) Is language learning really a female affair? *Language Learning Journal* 1 (1), 40–43.

Maccoby, E. (ed.) (1966) *The Development of Sex Differences*. London: Tavistock.

Preuschoff, G. (2004) *Raising Girls*. London: Thorsens.

Slaby, R.G. and Frey, K.S. (1975) Development of gender consistency and selective attention to same-sex models. *Child Development* 46, 849–856.

Tannon, D. (1990) *You Just Don't Understand: Women and Men in Conversation*. New York, NY: William Morrow & Co.

Warrington, M., Younger, M. and Williams, J. (2000) Student attitudes, image and the gender gap. *British Educational Research Journal* 26 (3), 393–407.

Williams, M., Burden, R. and Lanvers, U. (2002) 'French is the language of love and stuff': Student perceptions of issues related to motivation in learning a foreign language. *British Educational Research Journal* 28 (4), 503–528.

Note: You can read more about the families of Gerry, Christina, Lilian, Claudia, Jenifer, Toni, Nadya, Josie, Odile, Alice & Vicky and Lisa in *Family Profiles* at the end of the book.

Chapter 6
Birth Order: A Child's Position in the Family

This chapter looks at birth order, one of the factors which may affect bilingualism in the family. Birth order is the position of the child in the family – first-born, second-born, middle-born or last-born. Each order can be linked to a type of character or personality. The first part of this chapter investigates what birth order is, and what effect it could have on children's emerging language skills. There is also the issue of parents judging their children by their position in the family and the subtle differences in parenting as the family grows.

The second part of this chapter looks at some of the bilingual families that we heard about in Chapter 1 along with data from families that I interviewed via the survey and case studies. I asked the bilingual and multilingual families what effect birth order had on their children. Was there a difference between the first, middle or their last children's language use? Which child had the widest vocabulary use, the most correct or the most imaginative language skills? Could birth order affect bilingualism within the home? We hear the parent's thoughts on their children and their position in the family.

FIRST-BORN, MIDDLE-BORN OR LAST-BORN CHILDREN

Each child's position in the family is known as their birth order, for example, first-born, second-born, middle-born or last-born. Birth order has been linked to personality types, for example, a serious and ambitious first-born, a curious and eager-to-please middle-born, or a rebellious and independent last-born child. In large families, of more than three children, the third or fourth child is referred to in the same way as the middle-born one. An only child without a sibling is often discussed as having similar personality traits to a first-born. Siblings with a large age gap (e.g. five to

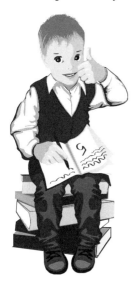

seven years apart) are usually considered in the same way as only children, because the effects of the other sibling on each child are weak. Here is a brief summary of personality traits associated with each child taken from several books on birth order (see the references at the end of the chapter). These birth-order personality traits are generalized and therefore do not apply to all children.

Psychologists are generally in agreement that the oldest child, regardless of gender, has an early advantage over the siblings. *First-born* and *only* children can be described as motivated, ambitious, responsible, anxious, critical, cautious and sensitive. They benefit from sharing a home with two interested adults who talk directly to him or her. The first-born child has a physical advantage, at least for a short time, until other siblings grow. First-borns tend to get better grades and are more likely to have a higher level of education, probably because they are more motivated to do what their parents and teachers ask of them. Parents often have high expectations for their first-borns. Consequently, first-born children may have high goals, adhere to rules or have higher anxiety levels compared to other siblings.

Second-born (or *middle-born* children of a large family) are described as easy-going, caring, curious, sociable and good at second guessing. They may benefit from having less pressure to please the parents. They can be more adventurous and less concerned about rules than their older siblings. Their parents feel more confident about parenting second time around. Second or middle-born children look up to their older sibling as a role-model, but they also might have to take care of the youngest sibling, playing simultaneous roles of teacher and pupil. Middle-born children may try hard to please everyone and sometimes end up being negotiators or go-betweens for the siblings. However, some psychologists note that middle-born children, sandwiched between an older and a younger sibling, lose out both ways, neither fussed over for the being the first or the last child.

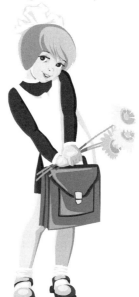

The *last-born* child has the role of being the 'baby' of the family. They are described as playful, cheerful, irresponsible, adventurous and rebellious. Last-born children may profit from the status of being the baby and the parental attention it gives them. As the baby of the family they are sometimes unintentionally spoilt by parents, and are the focus of parents' and siblings' attention while they are young. They may be more prone to throwing tantrums when things are not going their way, using emotional blackmail to get what they want or becoming easily discouraged when things do not go as they planned. They are sometimes prone to high anxiety and the need to negotiate for attention. Last-born children sometimes play the role of joker in the family.

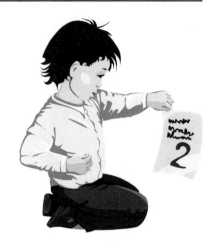

THE BIRTH ORDER DEBATE

Much research has been conducted on birth order, particularly over the last 40 years. Data on birth order is relatively easy to collect; while running other psychological tests researchers simply note the birth position of the interviewee and then align the results with a personality test. Several books are available on the subject concerning how, as adults and parents, we can make birth order work to our advantage. Anecdotes and generalized observations about first-, second- or last-born children, or adults, are frequently voiced within families or parenting groups about someone who behaves in a typically studious 'First-born' or babyish 'Last-born' manner. Does birth order exist or is it all just a myth? Understandably, only some of the birth order characteristics can be applied to children and many are refuted. Nevertheless, many psychologists agree that birth order can have an effect on how an individual learns to deal with life circumstances and relationships.

One of the first recorded comments on birth order came from British scientist Sir Frances Galton, cousin of Charles Darwin, and a famous botanist and writer on evolution. In the 1700s, Galton noticed that membership of the prestigious Royal Society in London had an exceptionally high number of first-born British scientists. In the 1970s, Stanford University psychologist Robert Zajonc studied birth order effects and concluded that both first-borns and last-born children get more attention from their parents and achieve higher academic scores than middle-born children. Zajonc also implied that first-borns have higher IQs than their siblings, an issue that raises several questions about how we judge or acquire intelligence. It is most likely that the recorded IQ gains were due to the age difference between siblings, or siblings choosing to excel in different areas, like art or sport, which are not always valued in a formal written IQ test. It could also be that parents tend to rate their first-born child as more intelligent, because he or she is older than the others and therefore involved in more challenging academic studies. But the myth persists that first-borns are the clever, bright members of the family in the media. For example, an article on birth order in *Time* magazine (November 12, 2007) reported on the high number of first-born members of Congress and surgeons and a UK *Times* (April 12, 2008) article was titled *'Older and Wiser: Why first-born children have higher IQ's'*.

Conversely, Dr Frank Sulloway (*Born To Rebel – Birth Order, Family Dynamics and Creative Lives*, 1997), science historian and research scholar at the Massachusetts Institute of Technology, thought that younger siblings have more to gain intellectually from their birth position. Sulloway combed through biographies and published scientific works of famous later-born scientists, leaders or revolutionary figures, such as Charles Darwin, Galileo, Benjamin Franklin and Voltaire. He described the propensity of the later, or the last-born, members of a family to be 'rebellious' and make great discoveries. Charles Darwin was the fifth of a family of seven and was the perfect example of a later-born child who changed the world with his revolutionary thoughts on evolution. Sulloway contrasts first and later-born children, saying,

> It is natural for firstborns to identify more strongly with power and authority. They arrive first in the family and employ their superior size and strength to defend their special status. Relative to their younger siblings, firstborns are more assertive, socially dominant, ambitious, jealous of their status, and defensive. As underdogs within the family system, some younger siblings are inclined to question the status quo and in some cases develop a "revolutionary personality". In the name of revolution, laterborns have repeatedly challenged the time-honored assumptions of their day. From the ranks have come the bold explorers, the iconoclasts, and the heretics of history. (Sulloway, 1997: xiv)

In a historical context, the families Sulloway discussed were large, often with 7–12 children, and typically the oldest son would stand to inherit the family property. Therefore, since they had no inheritance to look forward to, a younger son or daughter might have been more motivated to travel and search for a creative solution to finance their lifestyle or personal projects in science. Second- or later-born children in the 20th century may have less need to explore or change history. Judy Dunn and Robert Plomin (*Separate Lives: Why Siblings Are So Different*, 1990) compared famous sibling sets of writers, sportsmen, politicians and historical figures through their biographies. Dunn and Plomin concluded that birth order has very little effect, saying that siblings differ due to heredity and the way the parents treat them. They concluded that birth order simply '... plays only a bit part in the drama of sibling differences' (Dunn & Plomin, 1990: 85).

Swiss psychologists, Cécile Ernst and Jules Angst (1983) made a comprehensive review of all the research on birth order from 1946 to 1980, which amounted to nearly a thousand publications in all. Ernst and Angst also surveyed 7582 young students in Zurich about their sibling experiences. After assessing all evidence, Ernst and Angst concluded that birth order was simply not an important factor at all. Most of the research was either badly designed or biased. By not 'controlling' or allowing for the effect of social class on family size, the studies were not giving a true picture of causes. When they eliminated studies which lacked class or family size controls, they still could not find any significant effects. Ernst and Angst recommended that researchers stop looking for birth order effects and look elsewhere. Judith Rich Harris (*The Nurture Assumption*, 1998) thought that genetics, heredity and society play a greater role. Judith Rich Harris said that researchers simply kept on analyzing and reanalyzing their data until they found something on birth order that they could prove. Judith made the pertinent point that the strongest 'proof' of birth order is seen when parents judge their children (i.e. 'Our son is a typical first-born'.) Therefore, the most statistically significant results were usually found when the *parents* or *siblings* commented on family members in a home situation. This parent–child view on birth order could be an internal way to categorize and compare family members. The way parents deal with each child, according to their birth order, could show some subtle differences in parenting. Birth order could be the parent's way of dealing with each child individually, rather than the children fitting their birth-order profile.

Parents can follow established patterns of behavior linked to a child's place in the family. For example, Judy Dunn (*Sisters and Brothers*, 1985) observed how second-time parents often went from 'rigidity' to 'flexibility', over issues such as eating, bedtime or habits like sucking a thumb, having a pacifier/dummy or a comfort object (a special toy or cloth). In many cases this is done unconsciously and without any discussion between the parents. Judy Dunn voices the experiences of many parents, saying,

> It is widely held that parents are more easygoing and relaxed with their later-born children, and that first-borns are more difficult to cope with. (Dunn, 1990: 92)

This is most evident with a child's early language use. Beginning to talk is one of the great milestones of childhood development, along with walking and sleeping through the night. Parents can invest a lot of time and effort into helping their child learn their language. Naturally, this can be a distinct advantage for the first child. The first child is somewhat of a 'test-run' for parents, unless parents have had a lot of experience working or caring for a young child. Parents try to do things 'right' and establish certain rules and routines which they are strict about, especially with the first child. An older sibling is often asked to behave in a more responsible and serious manner, either helping with the care of younger siblings or keeping busy while the parents are occupied. Perhaps first-borns get the label 'responsible' simply because their parents decide for them that they must be. Arriving in a more lenient and permissive environment, a later-born child can profit from more relaxed parenting. Later-born children are often treated much more indulgently by the parents and other family members than their older siblings. They are able to 'get away' with more, or adapt family rules. Researchers Judy Dunn and Carol Kendrick (*Siblings: Love, Envy & Understanding*, 1982) observations on sibling pairs in Cambridge found that mothers typically favored the youngest one, especially in arguments where older brothers were often punished unfairly. Older siblings were three times more likely to be scolded or punished (even when they did not do anything).

Whether the first, second or last child stands to gain, or lose, from their position is a rather gray area. Thus, there are opposing viewpoints and it is difficult to agree on *which* birth order positions are advantageous and whether they affect personality. Birth order certainly exists within sibling sets, but it is still questionable as to whether it actually has an effect. The stereotyping of oldest, middle and last children with regard to their birth order and personality traits is harmless, as long as we recognize it.

> *Birth order* is a debatable issue. However, many psychologists think a child's place in the family can affect their behavior and attitude to life. Birth order is also linked to established societal patterns of how parents see the role of each layer of their family.

BIRTH ORDER AND LANGUAGE USE WITHIN THE BILINGUAL FAMILY

Language is very important in the bilingual family and patterns can exist in the way parents react to each child's speech in their family. Second-born children arrive in a home where parents are used to talking to children. Colin Baker (*A Parents' and Teachers' Guide to Bilingualism*, 2007) comments on birth order:

> When the second child arrives, the language pattern of the household tends to be relatively well established. With the second birth, decisions about language interaction in the home have already been established. The language the first-born child speaks to each parent will have been standardized, with the likelihood that younger children will follow a similar pattern. (Baker, 2007: 51)

In the bilingual family, the second-born child will usually fit in with the 'pattern of language interaction' already up and running in the household. The younger siblings could benefit from parents who have some experience with bilingualism and have a model to follow. There has been very little research done on the connection between birth order and language skills, and even less on birth order and bilingualism. We know that in bilingual families where English is the dominant language, in a monolingual country, and the parents are maintaining a minority or heritage language at home, the later-born children tend to learn English at an earlier age than their older brothers and sisters (see Fishman, 1991; Wong-Fillmore, 1991). One recent interesting study in America showed the shift from heritage to majority language within the family. Sarah Shin (*Developing in Two Languages: Korean Children in America*, 2005) observed Korean heritage families living in America, focusing on the shift to English in their households. Sarah surveyed 204 families with children aged 4–18 years, recording their birth position and their level of bilingualism. She recorded that 79% of the first-born children spoke both Korean and English and 66% of the second-born children. However, only 43% of the third-born children had acquired both languages. Over time the parents spoke less Korean too, and the household moved from a *minority-language-at-home* strategy to a mixed language one. The first-born child appeared to be an important factor in the sibling's language use too as Sarah commented in her 2002 paper,

> As later-born children learn from their elder siblings to value English as the language of power, they are at the same time discouraged from speaking the native language. (Shin, 2002: 109).

Sarah found that the young siblings in her study of 12 Korean/American sibling sets were often ridiculed or repeatedly corrected by older siblings when they spoke Korean. Consequently this led to a 'vicious cycle', with the younger ones choosing not to speak Korean in front of the older siblings, and less active language use in Korean over time.

Here is a fictionalized example of how parents might treat each child according to their birth order. It is generalized, and does not apply to all parents or children.

The first or only bilingual child

The new parents are truly amazed to hear the child babble a few syllables in each language, and eventually speak their first words. Each parent is sure he can hear his or her language first and praises the child frequently. The parents each listen carefully to the child's somewhat limited speech, translating if needs be. The parents note the words along with the first mixed dual language sentences. There is a lot of 'adult-to-child' conversation and explanations of the world around them in both languages. Parents make an effort to speak clearly and repeat mispronounced words back to the child. They frequently correct and try to improve the child's way of speaking with explanations.

But the parents can be overambitious if their child does not hit developmental milestones on time, or is not speaking as well as a child of the same age. Worry often sets in around age two, when the neighbor's monolingual kid is talking in paragraphs. They often ask for external guidance or speech therapy if they feel that the child is not talking properly. The parents usually follow a language strategy and discuss their goals for their child's future multilingualism.

Parents typically say: 'Do you know the word for this?'

The second or middle bilingual child

Secure in the knowledge that their child will speak both languages at some point the parents relax a little. They may make some notes or write down amusing expressions, but not with the fervor of the first-born. If the child is not speaking both languages by age three they might seek help, otherwise they do not worry too much, even if one language takes some time to become actively used. When the first child is out at school or with friends, the parents talk more to the second child.

The second, or middle-child, benefits from playing and practicing languages with their siblings. He or she listens in to conversations at home and may surprise them all by knowing more than they thought for their age. Parents are less concerned about proper language use, and often the sibling will correct the younger one for them. They might try to improve any obviously wrong or ungrammatical speech, then leave the rest to teachers and time. Parents still follow the same strategy; unless it did not work with the first child. The children decide between themselves which language they prefer to use, most typically the language of the country or school where they spend most of their time, or a mix of their languages.

Parents typically say: 'Go and play with your sister/brother!'

The last-born bilingual child

Parents are sure that the new baby will talk this time around and language use is a joint effort, shared between parents and siblings. The older siblings delight in teaching the youngest ones essential words in both languages and playing teacher/pupil games with him or her. The older ones might read or sing to the little one and try to encourage his or her developing vocabulary. When the others are away at school or with friends the parents chat along to the third child, but often while doing something else.

Like the second and middle children the baby gets to listen in to adults talking to children, and older children talking to their peer friends; and quickly learns what makes people pay attention. The last-born child is often good at second – guessing what people want to hear, and can make jokes. But he or she might use screaming tantrums or employ baby talk to get attention too. Language patterns are well established and mixing may increase in families where all members are fluently bilingual. The children make the decision on which language to use together and with the new siblings, which may be a mix of two or more languages or more typically the language of the country/school.

Parents typically say: 'Who taught the baby that word?'

First-borns can excel linguistically and may use more of the minority language initially with parents. *Second-, middle-* or *last-born* children may be exposed earlier to the majority language or the language of school.

VOCABULARY AND LANGUAGE USE LINKED TO BIRTH ORDER

In Chapter 1 we looked at some biographical case studies by parent-linguists. Most of the first children appeared to be serious about fluently speaking two languages and keen to please their parents. In the Leopold family in America, the older daughter,

Hildegard, was a precocious early English/German bilingual with an accurate knowledge of both languages. We see the same pattern in the Fantini family, also in America, where their first-born son, Marco, was speaking both Spanish and English fluently at an early age. In the Saunders home in Australia, the first-born son, Frank, considered himself fully bilingual in German and English, compared to the other two children. In the multilingual environment of the Tokuhama-Espinosa family, the first-born daughter, Natalie, was described as being very articulate for her age. However, it is not only the first child who shines linguistically. In the Cunningham-Andersson family of four English/Swedish children, the second child, Anders, was considered by his parents to be the most fluent in both languages. These examples taken from academic studies are from families where one or both of the parents had a linguistic background or profession. Is the first-born naturally better at languages than the younger siblings? Did the international families I surveyed perceive that the first-born child had an advantage? I asked parents to agree or disagree with the statement:

Is the first-born child likely to be the most successful at becoming bilingual?

Just over half of the parents (57%) from the survey disagreed or disagreed strongly with the statement that being a first-born was an advantage to being bilingual (Figure 6.1). On the other hand, only 21% of the parents agreed that being the first child would help a child become successful at speaking two languages. One in five parents said that they were not sure. Could there be a difference in terms of language skills between the first and later-born children? Studies on monolingual children suggest this. A first child with motivated parents and more time for language input might have a wider vocabulary. This could lead to first-born children having a more 'correct' or 'proper' way of speaking to please their parents. We might expect the first child to also have a wider overall vocabulary due to the extra time they spend alone with the parents, before a sibling joined the family. There might be more time for parents to spend time with the first child reading or writing. Perhaps later-born children would have a more varied and 'creative' speech, having had more input and variety from both

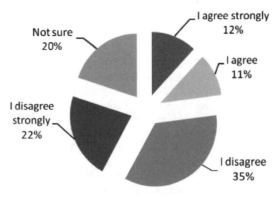

Figure 6.1 *Is the first-born child likely to be the most successful at becoming bilingual?*

parents and siblings. Second- or later-born children often have better conversational skills, and are quicker at understanding what people are talking about or guessing hidden meanings. Perhaps later-born children would be more creative with both languages than their older siblings? Did the online survey parents find a difference of language use depending on their children's birth order? To find out more about the language skills of first, second and last-born children I asked the families in the survey a series of questions on whether they saw a difference in each of their children, relating to their children's knowledge of vocabulary, their effort to speak in a correct way and creativity.

109	First-born
98	Second-born
17	Third-born

I first asked the 105 parents to consider their own children's overall vocabulary, according to their age, and answer the following questions.

Allowing for age, which of your children has the widest vocabulary?

Parents were encouraged to choose only one child, but in some cases parents chose two children, so I had 114 replies for this question, from 105 parents (Figure 6.2). For this question, nearly 90% of the 105 parents rated their first child as having the widest vocabulary use. For 25% of the parents, it was the second children who had the widest vocabulary and just three chose the third child. The low count of three third-born children would be expected since there were only 17 in the study. However, there were similar numbers of first-borns (109) and second-born children (98). This does show that, in the parent's eyes, the first-born child does have a verbal advantage over his or her siblings. But does the first child have the same advantage in both languages? I asked the parents to judge their children in terms of their total language skills.

Allowing for age, which of your children has the widest vocabulary in all their languages added together?

Interestingly, the results from this second question were almost identical to the first question (Figure 6.3). Eighty-nine percent of the 105 parents rated their first child

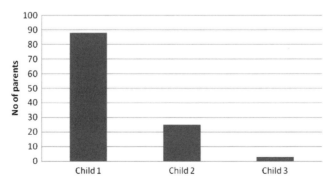

Figure 6.2 Widest vocabulary use

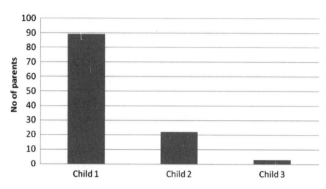

Figure 6.3 Widest vocabulary use in all languages

as having the widest bilingual knowledge, along with 22% second-born children and just three third-born children. This shows that the majority of first children were able to transfer their strong knowledge of vocabulary across to both languages. First-borns benefited from a higher linguistic score not only in one, but perhaps in two (or three languages in trilingual families). Whether this is due to their early exposure to adult conversations, or more one-to-one parent talk, or to typically first-born determination and curiosity is hard to say. What we can agree on is that the majority of parents see their first child as the one who has learned more words and expressions than the other children. But is the child with the widest vocabulary levels also the most correct speaker in the family? Does the first-born know his grammatical rules too? This was the next question for the parents.

Would there be a difference between siblings in the way they manipulated language? Which child would have the most 'correct' way of communicating in terms of parental perceptions? For example, following established grammatical norms or conventions of speech and writing in each language. The first child has a good reason to communicate with adults and often gets much praise and encouragement. In such an adult-orientated world there is likely to be more emphasis on speaking properly. Would a first-born try harder to use the right language with the appropriate person? I asked the parents:

Allowing for age, which of your children has the most 'correct' language use?

Like in the previous questions on vocabulary use, the first-born child was judged as the one who speaks most correctly by 77% of the 105 parents. Twenty-three percent of the parents thought that the second-born child was most correct one in their family (Figure 6.4). Five parents chose their third-born child as the most correct one too. This shows that in the majority of families the first-born child not only has a wide vocabulary, but also uses language in the right way, as perceived by his or her parents. The final question I asked the parents was related to creative use of language. Would the first-child outshine the others in terms of imaginative use of language too? Which child

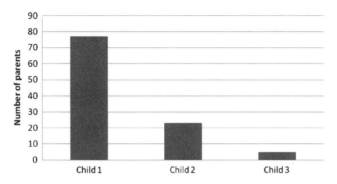

Figure 6.4 Most correct language use

in the family would use language in a more creative, or communicative way? Middle children are often described in birth order books, and by parents, as the 'translator' or diplomat of the family. They are known for their communication skills and making others feel at ease. Who are the creative ones in the family? I asked the parents:

Allowing for age, which of your children uses language most imaginatively?

First-borns scored well, but second-born children had a higher count than before. In the study 63% of the parents thought that their first child was the most imaginative (Figure 6.5). Thirty-six percent of the parents considered that the second child was the creative one. Six parents rated their third child as the one having the most imagination. Perhaps the second-born children or last-born children see language more as a tool for imagination than for correct proper language use. A second-born child needs to communicate not only with his or her parents, but also with their siblings. For child-to-child talk, a lively imagination is needed for sharing stories, rhymes and jokes.

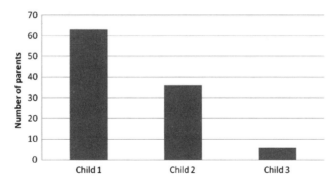

Figure 6.5 Most imaginative use of language

DOES BIRTH ORDER MAKE A DIFFERENCE?

Child one is more verbally proficient in nearly every area, though child two is making great progress, but on a slower time table.

Child one is much better at learning new languages, though child two is more literary and imaginative in English.

The second one speaks more clearly than the first one did at the same age.

The second one spoke much earlier and seems more comfortable switching

What did the case-study parents think about birth order? Several parents replied that birth order was just not relevant to their family. Nevertheless, there were some interesting comments from eight parents on the subject of birth order on their firstborn's strong effect on the language preferences the siblings had at home. In line with Sarah Shin's findings, there was a common theme of the first child 'setting' the language for the other children. An older more articulate child influenced younger siblings to choose one language over another as their preferred language. Josie, a trilingual mother, remarked that birth order had played an important role in the linguistic choices her children made. Their firstborn son, Niklas, made the decision to speak German with his two brothers, in an English language environment. This choice of inter-sibling language probably helped the family in supporting and maintaining German at home.

I think birth order affects bilingualism only to the extent that the eldest sibling probably determines which language is dominant. In our family, Niklas started at around age 6 to speak German almost all the time to me even though I would carry on in English. This was despite the fact that we were living then in an English-speaking environment and he had to communicate with many people in English. As soon as Tobias could speak German about as well as he could English, Niklas spoke German only to him. And both Niklas and Tobias now speak only German to Lukas.
Josie: Chinese/German/English trilingual family in Germany, mother of Niklas (12), Tobias (8) and Lukas (4)

Gerry, a Canadian mother of four bilingual children, also thought that the oldest child is a strong role model for bilingualism, and a bilingual first-born increases the odds of having bilingual siblings too. She makes the point that it can be easier for younger bilingual siblings, as they are already part of a 'group' and may not feel different or embarrassed about being bilingual in public.

If the first-born child is, or becomes, bilingual I think chances are good that subsequent children will be exposed to, offered or provided with the same opportunities. Younger siblings may even have an easier or much richer exposure to dual language use and thus, have an easier time being or becoming bilingual among the group.

Gerry: English/Spanish in Canada (OPOL), mother of four children (aged 13, 11, 7 and 5)

Comments on second children reported that many second children were 'better' than the first one, often to the parent's surprise. They were more 'comfortable' about being bilingual, liked playing with languages or language games. They benefited from their older siblings and the wider scope for practice. Martina, a Venezuelan mother married to an Italian, is introducing her daughters to English, alongside the two parental languages. Martina thinks that the second child has an advantage, thanks to the parents being more relaxed, and the second one being able to listen in to the first child talking.

Regarding birth order, I think that the second child is 'better' than the first one. We as parents feel at ease better with the second one than with the first one, where everything is new to us. When our first child, Alessia, was born I was the only one who spoke Spanish to her. But when Gaia was born she was able to watch since day one my interaction with Alessia. In fact, Gaia never mixed up Italian and Spanish, and has even corrected me when I have 'slipped' a word in Italian to my husband. She always says. "No, you say it like this …." I believe that the second one is able to have both languages in an easier way. Ever since Gaia started talking she always spoke in Spanish … something that Alessia never did.
Martina: Spanish/Italian/English trilingual family in Italy, mother of Alessia (8) and Gaia (6)

Like Martina, Alice is bringing up her two children with three languages and was worried that she could not give her second child the same language input as she did with her first-born daughter. However, the second child has benefited and gained more from being second in the family.

I used to think that I spent more time with my first-born, interacting more with her, speaking more with her than with my youngest one, and that as a result she got a lot more language-input from me than I was able to offer my younger son. I then realized that my daughter is playing a lot with her little brother – in English! So in the end he is actually exposed to a lot more language variety than when my daughter was his age. Isabella had 'only' us as language models, whereas Dominick is getting English from the parents and his sibling. I think that probably the more members there are in the family, and the more the kids interact with each other, the more this helps cement their bilingualism!
Alice: German/Spanish/English in Austria (Lingua Franca) mother of Isabella (5) and Dominick (2)

Fabiana found that birth order and language skills were different in her family of three girls and one boy. The first-born, Martine, excels at grammar and vocabulary, whereas her younger sister, third-born, Arianna is better at reading and writing in Italian (her mother's language).

All three girls are fluent in both languages, but it seems that Martina has a wider vocabulary than the sisters. In fact her Italian is much better than many Italian kids of her age, even though we visit Italy once a year. Natalia and Arianna's Italian is less grammatically correct than Martina's. We noticed that as soon as they step outside home their social language becomes English. They stopped using Italian among themselves as they used to and it became harder for Arianna to speak it. We have been sticking to OPOL and Arianna slowly managed to develop a very good Italian along with her English. They are now slowly learning to write and read Italian and in this case the birth order is reversed, in fact Arianna has a better grasp of the Italian phonetic and spelling, Natalia follows immediately after and Martina instead tends to apply English phonetics to it.

Fabiana: Italian/Chinese/English trilingual family in Malaysia, mother of Martina (10), Natalia (9), Arianna (6) and Thomas (1)

The parent's opinions show the variety of thoughts on birth order. The first child may have some advantage in 'setting' the language, through the status of being oldest and having a wider vocabulary. Middle and younger children may benefit from parents being less strict about language development, and older siblings who teach and model language use.

SUMMARY

We can see that birth order is useful as a general way of classifying each child's position in the family. There are some common personality traits of first-, second-, middle- or last-born children which both parents and researchers appear to agree on. First-born children tend to be seen as being more responsible, and younger ones appear to have less pressure and more freedom. This could affect children's developing language use and the way they communicate with adults and children. There is still an ongoing debate over whether the first- or later-born children gain in the long run. Nevertheless, it does seem apparent that there can be a subtle difference in treatment from the parents, in terms of the attention, interest and effort made developing child's language skills. This is natural in many ways, as the family evolves to encompass more personalities and needs. Parents may subconsciously reinforce birth order positions themselves, expecting more of the older child or giving more allowance to the younger ones. Some children may also be more affected by being displaced by another sibling or be more sensitive to the reduction in parental attention which could affect their immediate language use.

Birth order is not a strong factor in bilingual development, but it seems that first-born children could have a certain advantage over their younger siblings. Their speech is generally more correct and they appear to have a broader vocabulary in both languages. First-borns seem to care more about getting it right, which could make them naturally more suited to strict language strategies such as OPOL or *minority-language-at-home*, which demand a clear separation of languages and following rules on who speaks which language. The first-born does appear to control or influence the language patterns of the younger siblings. Parents agreed that a second or later-born can benefit from a sibling's experience. The younger siblings have possibly less direct one-to-one time with their parents, but gain from having a wider range of language models within the home. Later-born children would be likely to copy language choices made by their older siblings. Being first, second or last in the family does not guarantee bilingualism, but it might affect the language choices made by brothers and sisters.

Birth order also interacts with the gender and character of each child. In Chapter 7 we take a look at the individual personality and personalities of the children. Can a child's natural tendency to be shy or chatty affect their language patterns? Is it better to be an extrovert or an introvert when learning two or more languages? Are some children 'naturally' good at languages? These questions will be looked at along with a rivalry between siblings and language friction.

Further reading on birth order

Baker, C. (2007) *A Parents' and Teachers' Guide to Bilingualism* (3rd edn). Clevedon: Multilingual Matters.

Dunn, J. (1985) *Sisters and Brothers: The Developing Child*. MA: Harvard University Press.

Dunn, J. and Kendrick, C. (1982) *Siblings: Love, Envy & Understanding*. MA: Harvard University Press.

Dunn, J. and Plomin, R. (1990) *Separate Lives: Why Siblings are So Different*. New York: Basic Books.

Ernst, C. and Angst, J. (1983) *Birth Order: Its Influence on Personality*. Berlin & New York: Springer-Verlag.

Fishman, J.A. (1989) *Bilingual Education: An International Sociological Perspective*. Clevedon: Multilingual Matters.

Galton, F. (1874) *English Men of Science*. London: Macmillan.

Harris, J.R. (1998) *The Nurture Assumption*. New York: W.W. Norton & Co.

Krohn, K.E. (2000) *Everything You Need to Know about Birth Order*. New York: Rosen.

Leman, K. (2001) *The Birth Order Connection*. MI: F.H. Revell.

Shin, S.J. (2002) Birth order and the language experience of bilingual children. *TESOL Quarterly* 36 (6), 103–113.

Shin, S.J. (2005) *Developing in Two Languages: Korean Children in America*. Clevedon: Multilingual Matters.

Sulloway, J.F. (1997) *Born to Rebel: Birth Order, Family Dynamics and Creative Lives*. New York: Vintage Books.

Time Magazine. (2007) *The Secrets of Birth Order*. November 12, 32–8.

The Times (UK) (2008) *Older and Wiser: Why First-born Children have Higher IQ's*. April 12, 4–5.

Wallace, M. (1999) *Birth Order Blues: How Parents Can Help their Children Meet the Challenges of Birth Order*. New York: Henry Holt & Co.

Wong Fillmore, L. (1991) When learning a second language means losing the first. *Early Childhood Research Quarterly* 6, 323–346.

Zajonc, R.B. (1976) Family configuration and intelligence. *Science* 192, 227–236.

Note: You can read more about the language patterns and families of Josie, Gerry, Martina, Alice and Fabiana in *Family Profiles* at the end of the book.

Chapter 7

Individual Differences: Same Languages, Different Language Histories

In this chapter we look at how the personality and experiences of each individual sibling might affect language use. Siblings living in the same home with the same parents can turn out to be more different than alike in character. One child can be confident, chatty and sociable, while another one is shy, timid or reluctant to talk. Why is there a difference between children being brought up in the same home? Is it linked to their genes, parental treatment or the home environment? Is it a question of nature or nurture? Each child has its own language history and each child in the family deals with its bilingualism in a different way. I asked the case study families and the surveyed parents about the individual differences they saw in their children.

Some children excel in languages, while others struggle. Within the same bilingual family one child might be 'brilliant', effortlessly picking up two or three languages, while another child strives to just communicate in one language. One child can feel more attached to one parent's language. Are there some personality traits that could affect language use? For example, does being an introvert or extrovert affect a child's chances of learning or using two or more languages? In some families there may be sibling rivalry or competition between siblings, a friction in which language is implicated. One might try to block other children from using a certain language. Siblings might tease or laugh at other siblings when they make mistakes or have the wrong accent. We hear what the case-study families and academic researchers thought about these debatable issues.

THE NATURE OR NURTURE DEBATE

Over the last 40 years, psychologists and child development researchers have investigated the link between a child's personality, home environment and the way the child is brought up by his or her parents. A child's personality can affect the way it relates emotionally to other people and the way it behaves. There are children who are shy or scared of new experiences in life, whereas other children are keen to socialize and try new things. Some babies are smiley and enjoy being played with while other babies pull away and avoid physical contact. In school some children love being social and playing with other children, while others find the dynamics of a classroom situation or making friends overwhelming. The question of the parent's role in a child's developing personality remains a heated debate, mainly because parents are often implicated when a child has problems. This is often referred to as the 'parent–child' effect (see Alexander Thomas, 1968), who proposed the idea of 'goodness of fit' in parent–child relationships).

In theory, parents should be aware of each child's character and deal with it appropriately. They should try to 'fit' to their children and react accordingly to their personality. The subject of how parents affect their children is commonly discussed in parenting books and magazines, with parents often being blamed for not helping their children more. However, even with the best parenting skills most families find they have one child who they find 'difficult' at some stage. Some children have a way of behaving which the parents do not like or approve of, such as screaming for attention or having a tantrum. Families with two or more children in the same home with the same parenting patterns can have children with different personalities. Are the parents to blame when their children do not turn out as they expected? Judy Dunn, a child psychologist, and Robert Plomin, an expert in behavioral genetics (*Separate Lives: Why Siblings Are So Different*, 1990), investigated the relationship between genes and the environment. Dunn and Plomin calculated that siblings share only between 30% and 50% of inherited parental genes. These genes could manifest themselves in a *tendency* to be happy, angry, aggressive or kind to other people. This means parents and siblings share some common family personality traits, such as kindness or anger, but not necessarily all of them. That is why two children living in the same home with the same parents can turn out quite differently. Children adopted into a family often have as much in common with their adopted parents as their biological siblings. Parents and the shared home environment do play a role in the development of a child, but there is still an unexplained area of nonshared individual experiences. Using data from several wide-ranging longitudinal studies in Cambridge, England and Colorado, America, Dunn and

Plomin found that only 15% of the shared genes accounted for personality traits. This implies that there can be a 'difference' of 85% within siblings. Steven Pinker (*The Blank Slate*, 2002) discussed the nature/nurture debate and explained the differences,

> The **shared** environment is what impinges on us and our siblings alike: our parents, our home life, and our neighborhood. The **non-shared** or **unique** environment is everything else: anything that impinges on one sibling but not another, including parental favoritism (Mom always liked you best), the presence of the other siblings, unique expectations. (Pinker, 2002: 378)

Setting aside the inherited genes and the effect of the shared home environment, Judy Dunn and Robert Plomin concentrated on investigating the 85% of *non-shared* factors that make siblings different. They wondered if the wide sibling difference was linked to the way the parents treated each child. In the Colorado study siblings, aged from 12 months to 3 years old, were recorded in natural situations playing and talking to their mother. Their results showed that the mothers treated the children in the same way at each age. The level of attention, fussing or interaction the mothers engaged in with each sibling did not vary over time. However, the other sibling who was closely watching often thought *he* or *she* was being treated differently. Some siblings felt that their mother was paying more attention to the younger one, even though the mother fussed over them in the same way when they were at the same age. This shows that siblings are very much aware of how the family unit operates at a young age, and how each person is treated individually. This presumes a much more complicated situation than the 'parent–child' theory. Siblings are not only sensitive to how their parents treat each child, but how each child gets treated too. Dunn and Plomin observed,

> … children are sensitive to not only to how their parents relate to them, but also to how their parents relate to their siblings, and that children monitor and respond to that other relationships just as they monitor the relationship between their parents. (Dunn & Plomin, 1990: 79)

Judith Rich Harris (*The Nurture Assumption*, 1998) also argues that parents are not responsible for forming their child's personality. Each child finds a different way to fit in to his or her world and parents naturally treat them differently because of this. Judith calls this the 'child-to-parent' effect and says,

> As most parents realize shortly after the birth of their second child, children come into this world already different from each other. Their parents treat them differently because of their different characteristics. (Harris, 1998: 27)

She strongly disputes the theory that parenting or nurturing has a long-lasting effect on the child. Judith concludes that the child's inherited genetic makeup interacts with their parents, siblings, friends and peers. Inherited traits like kindness can be enriched with the right social group, or aggression and anger can grow in an environment which encourages violence. The child wants to 'fit in' or align with his or her social group rather than with the parents. Naturally, parents still have a role to play in forming their child's characters, and are implicated in choosing where they live and their school, but they are not wholly responsible. The 'socialization' of the child, within his or her own peer group, is what creates sibling differences. The sensitive and complex interaction between children's genes, environment, parents' treatment and potential inter-sibling conflict is difficult to predict.

> Even after *sharing* a close home environment, siblings can be different. In a family with two or more children, the siblings could turn out to have quite different personalities. As parents we treat each child differently too, perhaps without even being aware of it.

LANGUAGE ACQUISITION

Babies acquire language in a relatively short time of a few years. Do we learn to speak instinctively, in the same way we learn to walk, or are we taught by our parents? The way young children learn to speak has been the subject of much research in the field of linguistics since the 1960s. One of the instigators of this research was the American philosopher and academic, Noam Chomsky, now Professor of Linguistics at the Massachusetts Institute of Technology, who considered the issue of how children 'acquire' a language from a different perspective. Chomsky (*Language and Mind*, 1968) described how a child is 'programmed' to speak over the first few years of development. A child's acquisition of language is automatic and all children follow a similar pattern. Their speech starts with babbling and sounds, moves on to producing familiar nouns, short two- or three-word sentences before becoming fully grammatical in less than six years. Chomsky called his theory the Universal Grammar, because the same pattern of development is repeated in all languages. This theory was revolutionary in that it explained that language is a genetically endowed trait and parents do not 'teach' their children how to speak. Parents certainly encourage and enrich their children's speech, but the emerging language development we see in early childhood appears to be a preset innate instinct.

In a bilingual family the emergence of two languages can be witnessed *simultaneously*, especially in OPOL homes where each parent speaks a different language. In other families a child can learn a second language *sequentially*, after mastering a first language (usually after age three or four). In this situation the parents often report that this second language is learnt from the community, the school and friends. This innate capacity to mimic the people around the child is best shown by the way children quickly pick up their friend's accent or local slang from the school playground. The social influence is seen clearly in children who move to a country using a different language. In immigrant families with children, the parents are not even needed for the children to pick up a new language. Academic Steven Pinker (*The Blank Slate*, 2002), the son of an immigrant family who came to live in America, made the valid point that children do not only copy their parents. He says,

> People's accents almost always resemble the accents of their childhood peers, not the accents of their parents. Children of immigrants acquire the language of their adopted homeland perfectly, without a foreign accent, as long as they have access to native speaking peers. They then try to force their parents to switch to the new language, and if they succeed, they may forget the mother tongue entirely. (Pinker, 2002: 391)

This illustrates that even though the parents might 'facilitate' language, it is the wider community and the children's friends who bring the language to life. The same scenario is seen in families all around the world who move to a new country with a different language with young children. These children quickly pick up the language of the country, often with very little help from their parents. Thus, there is an interaction between a genetic 'blueprint' and the child's environmental experiences. Nevertheless, as Steven Pinker rightly points out, the fear of many immigrant families is that their children will lose their home or heritage language as social pressure forces the children to prefer the new country language. Can parents persuade a child to use a certain language? Generally, case studies illustrate that the country/school language (or majority language) dominates the minority language, no matter how much the parents want their child to continue speaking it. Many bilingual families report on how their children refuse to use a home or parental language outside the home. In the Caldas French/English household, the home language (French) was carefully monitored for the three children, to the exclusion of English-language television. Vacations were in French-language Québec, where the parents enrolled the children in French-language camps or local schools. Nevertheless, by adolescence the children were noticeably more affected by their peer group. As Stephen recounts,

> Thus after approximately age 11, it was the children's peer groups and not we, the parents, that furthered and perfected our project goal of rearing perfectly fluent bilingual children. (Caldas, 2006: 191)

Even the children of two linguist parents, who may have inherited excellent linguistic genes, do not always become gifted multilinguals. It is the unique mix of genes, home environment and each child's own personal experiences which create each linguistic pattern; a mix which is more evident than ever in dual-language or multilingual households. Parents have a role to play in offering practice, encouragement and sustaining bilingualism over time. But friends or peers language use can possibly affect the child's language use more than the parents, so parents may need to be aware of their child's social world and the languages used outside the home.

> Children acquire *language patterns* both from their parents and society. The peer group can have a strong effect.

DIFFERENT LANGUAGE HISTORIES

I felt closer to my daughter because she speaks my language well and we can discuss and chat together more. My son makes a little effort when he has to, but that's it.

Our oldest child had delayed speech, limited knowledge of vocabulary, and her sentences were simplistic. The second one talked all the time!

We did the same thing with each child, but the last one hardly ever speaks both languages.

> *Jules*, 10, loves languages. In his Spanish-English household in Texas he takes all the chances he can to practice. Jules loves to chat to his mum's Spanish-speaking friends when they come round for coffee. He likes to watch the Spanish television channels and read comics in Spanish. His parents are proud of him and his fourth-grade teacher, who is married to a Hispanic, praises him regularly for his language skills. Jules has a younger sister, who is 8.
>
> *Sabrina*, 8, refuses to speak Spanish, except with her mother and even then she mixes the languages to make what she calls 'Spanglish'. She prefers to dance and spends much of her time at the studio after school. At school she is average, and hides the fact that she is bilingual. After eight years of 'trying' to make their daughter bilingual the parents say that she is simply 'not good at languages'. Her passion is for dance and that is what she is interested in.

Language histories are the background to how a child becomes bilingual. As we have seen, children who have the same environment do not always grow up to have the same language use or affinity to both languages. The language history can encompass all the small experiences that make up a child's life; a holiday, a special friend, a favorite book or film which inspires them to think or learn. Even if the whole family has the same experiences some children will get more or less out of each situation. For example, children in a library all make very different choices, some choose a picture book, others a novel or a comic book. Frank Sulloway (*Born to Rebel: Birth Order, Family Dynamics and Creative Lives*, 1997) thought that each child has a place or 'niche' in the family. In ecological phraseology a niche is created when different species share the available resources within their environment, and each one must diversify to avoid fighting over food or space. Frank says that families are like mini 'ecosystems' and within the family each child needs to find a 'niche'. A niche for a sibling might be excellence in music, sport, art or languages. Sulloway explains,

> Siblings compete with one another in an effort to secure physical, emotional, and intellectual resources from parents. Depending on differences in birth order, physical traits, and aspects of temperament, siblings create differing roles for themselves within the family system. (Sulloway, 1997: 21)

The niche theory could explain why some bilingual siblings are effortlessly fluent, while others struggle to communicate. There could there be an unspoken inter-sibling decision that one child may be less bilingual as a way to avoid rivalry with a verbally skilled sibling. In case studies on bilingual families, siblings appear to behave in different ways to each other in linguistic terms. They can embrace a language wholeheartedly or feel rather distant and unattached to one parental or country language. The most common difference is a scenario where one child found learning languages easy, while another sibling struggled, or one child feels more attached to one parental language. However, it is important to look at the whole family's circumstances, since one sibling may have had less input in one language or less chance to practice one language.

Xiao-lei Wang wrote about her two adolescent sons' trilingual development (*The Bilingual Family Newsletter*, 2009). As she encouraged their heritage language learning (Chinese) she commented on their different learning styles and how parents may want to consider their children's approach to language learning, saying,

> For example, my son Léandre is two years older than his brother Dominique. From a chronological perspective, I probably should set up higher Chinese learning goals and expectations for Léandre. However, in reality, I often do the opposite. This is simply because of Léandre's personality, and his tendency to avoid doing anything extra. Recently, while helping the children prepare for a Chinese examination, I asked Dominique to complete all the review materials in two hours and only asked Léandre to finish two of the exercises in the same amount of time. This disparity recognizes the disparity between my sons' personalities. (Wang, 2009: 3)

In some families one child may have more affinity with a parental culture and feel closer to them in cultural ways, enriching their language skills along the way. Leena Huss is a Finn who moved to live in Sweden with her Swedish husband. She described the linguistic progress of her three sons, now aged 29, 26 and 21 years old (*The Bilingual Family Newsletter*, 2003). In the beginning Leena spoke Finnish to her first and second children, and struggled to maintain her first language in an essentially monolingual climate. The family then moved to Finland when the boys were six and three, where they soon dropped their 'Swedish borrowings' and developed 'native fluency' in Finnish. Their third child was born in Helsinki and the family moved to Sweden when he was just a year old. To help support the minority language Leena asked her older sons to speak Finnish with the baby, which they did. As she says,

> In spite of the fact that the boys shared the same home environment and were exposed to the same kind of bilingual upbringing, they responded in different ways. Little brother, who was too young when we returned to Sweden to remember his time in Finland, eventually became the 'most Finnish' and would shout: 'Speak Finnish!' when he passed the bigger brothers' room and heard them speak Swedish with each other …

Leena remarks that this was accepted as the 'idiosyncrasy of the younger one', and his strong attitude to 'hold the Finnish flag high' helped maintain bilingualism and bicultural values in the home. A successful language strategy that worked with one child may not be suited to another child, as we saw in Chapter 2. Each child can react differently to their family languages and circumstances, and have differing motivations to speak each language. Meg Valenzuela, an American married to an Argentinean and living in Germany, wrote an article on balancing multilingual language use in families who move house frequently (*The Bilingual Family Newsletter*, 2004). Their first son, Lucas, was born in Germany and the couple strictly followed the OPOL + 1 approach, with success. The family then moved to Italy, and managed to maintain German through German-only weekends and German-speaking friends. When Lucas was six, the family returned to Germany and he settled in easily to the first grade of school. Their second son, Samuel, was born in Italy and had a different experience to his brother. His parents still spoke English and Spanish, as they had done with Lucas, but he was ambivalent toward German and had only a passive knowledge. Meg recounts,

> With our younger son, Samuel, we have walked a different path … Because of our good experience with the OPOL strategy, we chose to speak English and Spanish with him as we had with Lucas. We hoped that he would pick up enough German from our conversations with each other and Lucas … As a result, Samuel returned to Germany with a passive knowledge of German, but few experiences of using it actively

Samuel initially had problems settling into Germany, and struggled in comparison to his brother. Meg remarked that his German was much weaker than they expected. Searching for a way to help Samuel communicate more in German, the parents noticed that Samuel responded better to visual learning. He loved visiting the local library and looking at books. The parent's assumption that hearing German would be enough to support his bilingualism proved to be wrong for the second child. The story shows that we cannot assume that because our first child is good at languages the second child will be too, and the second child may not have the same learning patterns as the first one did.

> Even when parents bring up their children bilingual in the *same* way, the children can grow up with different *language histories*. One child may choose *not* to be bilingual or use one language.

LANGUAGE-GIFTED CHILDREN

Our daughter is more language-gifted

The eldest reads more and cares more for language so he is more accurate in its use

My daughter won't speak French, whereas her brother spoke fluently at the same age

Why are some children more gifted at languages than others? The parents can be mystified at the difference. They have followed the same language strategy, spoken the same languages and yet one child is fluent in both languages while the other one can barely make a sentence in one language. Assuming that one child does not have a serious speech impediment or learning disabilities, both children should have the same genetic ability to communicate. Children inherit a mix of their parents' genes, and usually in a bilingual family at least one parent is bilingual, so there is a chance that the children inherit a parental love of languages. The siblings have parents talking to them in the same languages, and have equal access to books, films and other materials in the family home. In theory, both children should stand a good chance at being multilingual.

Some children are outstanding linguists at a young age, like Hildegard Leopold and Mario Fantini, who were both preciously bilingual at a young age. These children seemed wired to communicate from a young age. Picking up two or more languages was easy and more of a game than a chore. Mario simply loved languages and was recorded as being fully bilingual at age two years and eight months. Not only did Mario speak Spanish, English and Italian at home, he also 'exhibited interest' in Japanese, German, Twi, Greek, Aymara and Quecha, all before he was 10 years old. This love of languages and a facility to switch languages certainly helped Mario become bilingual almost effortlessly. In the diary excerpts of Mario's speech between age three and four years old, his father commented,

> Throughout the diary a trend is clear. Mario showed increasing interest in the way people speak, in other ways to say things, and in other forms of language. He especially enjoyed linguistic play … He also enjoyed the custom of saying "good night" in five different ways: "Good night, buenas nochas, buona notte, boa noite, kali nicta," pointing to each of his fingers as he said each one. (Fantini, 1985: 48)

Like Mario, some children are fascinated by language as a whole, in communicating through speech, gestures, writing or reading. They like to 'play' with language and easily pick up accents and intonation. They are curious to learn more and practice with people they meet. These qualities are admirable and most of the bilingual families agreed that it was 'easier' to bring up such a child with two languages, and also, as one parent said about her daughter: 'It's so much easier for me, as a parent, to teach her, because she just loves anything to do with languages!' To find out whether the parents thought one child was better at languages I asked the case-study families:

Are some children naturally better at languages than others?

None of the case-study families themselves had experience of a particularly 'gifted' or talented child. In response to the question, the case-study families agreed that some children are naturally better at languages. Theresa mentioned that having a 'natural ear' for languages would benefit, in the way that some children can accurately mimic or copy a certain accent or sound. This would help the child to fit in and sound 'right'. Here are comments from Theresa, Alice, Martina and Odile.

> *I definitely think some kids are naturally better at languages than others. I think language abilities are like any other skill (musical ability, being good at math, etc.), and if you have a natural ear for learning languages, it'll be much easier for you to learn new languages than for people who don't.*
> Theresa: English/Spanish in Spain (OPOL), mother of Carmen (13), Rocio (11) and Violeta (9)

Alice also talked about the importance of experimenting and imitating languages. The ability to 'play' with language is also a useful skill that prepares children for the unpredictable nature of language. They are less likely to be put off when they have problems communicating and can try a different way of phrasing their words.

> *It seems as though some children have an easier time acquiring a language. It could be talent, or genes, or whatever! My daughter has encountered some obstacles during her language acquisition process, which my younger son doesn't seem to have. My son seems to speak, imitate, experiment a lot more with languages than my daughter ever did at his age.*
> Alice: German/Spanish/English in Austria (Lingua Franca) mother of Isabella (5) and Dominik (2)

Martina notes the importance of parental encouragement and incentives to keep language learning constant from an early age.

> *I believe that if a child is 'presented' a new language as early as possible, and that language is continuously present, he or she will be good at it. It's when there is no encouragement or constant incentive, that a child may become lazy in trying to speak that language.*
> Martina: Spanish/Italian/English trilingual family in Italy, mother of Alessia (8) and Gaia (6)

Odile, mother of three French/English children, comments on how the different personalities of her first- and second-born children contributed to their attitude toward language use at home with their mother.

> *I think my second child is actually 'better' at languages and I put it down to his personality rather than anything else. He likes things to be correct and not "messy" so he will correct himself and repeat in order to learn the right thing. My first one will repeat after me when I correct her without thinking about it but she's less curious, so she will keep on using the quickest way to express herself in French, even if it means using a few English words. As she knows I hate it and will always correct her she tends not to do that too often.*
> Odile: French/English (OPOL) family in Malaysia, mother of Amy (7), Luca (5) and Eliot (20 months)

The parents agreed that some kids are just gifted or talented at languages, like being good at art, music or sport. This is a bonus and can help them become fluently bilingual, but it should be noted that children also need motivation to speak languages and practice.

For some children, learning two or more languages is easy and fun. They appear to have an *'ear for languages'* and enjoy the challenge of becoming bilingual.

THE EXTROVERT MYTH

> *The older brother is simply more outgoing and loves to talk while younger sister likes to keep to herself more.*

> *Our daughter is quiet and reserved and will only speak if she knows what she will say is 'right', otherwise she'd rather say nothing.*

> *One kid loves learning new words, expressions or jokes; he tries them out on anyone who will listen!*

Extrovert	Introvert
Sociable	Can be shy
Outgoing	Quiet and reserved
Prefers to talk to someone than be alone	Prefers own company
Good at 'small talk' and starting chats	Can feel uncomfortable in social situations
Thinks best while talking	Thinks before speaking
Can be bored on their own	Can occupy time on their own easily

Would a child's attitude to life, and new situations, influence their communication skills? Parents and teachers often comment that a child who has a positive outgoing approach to life will have more opportunities to communicate with other people. Parents and teachers also agree that it is much easier to start a conversation with an extrovert chatty child than a shy reluctant one. A lively extrovert child can sustain a conversation. He or she might ask questions or engage in discussions, whereas a shy child might answer with brief 'yes' or 'no' to avoid prolonging the conversation. Quiet or introvert children might lack chances to practice languages, a particular concern to parents bringing up children with a minority language because practice is essential for fluency and development of a language. Kendall King and Alison Mackay (*The Bilingual Edge: Why, When and How to Teach Your Child a Second Language*, 2007) discussed personality in relation to children learning a second language, saying,

> For example, if your child is outgoing, she might seek out others more often for conversation and play; this in turn provides her with more exposure to the language and more opportunities to use the language. On the other hand, if your child is shy, she might be less likely to take risks and might have long silent or quiet periods when learning a second language. (King & Mackay, 2007: 87)

A sensitive child who cares what people think might be less willing to use a second language with strangers. Within a set of siblings there can be a subtle difference of one child being more 'chatty' or one being more reserved in their language use in certain environments. Would an extrovert child, have more chance of becoming bilingual? Charlotte Hoffmann described the individual approach to languages her two young children had,

> Christina is more sensitive, thoughtful and reserved than Pascual, and she still uses the appropriate language to each parent quite consistently … Pascual is more of an extrovert. From very early on he has always been keen to establish contact with new people and to be accepted by them. I feel this disposition may have helped him to overcome his linguistic shortcomings, which he was aware of and found frustrating. (Hoffmann, 1985: 489)

The link between personality and bilingual and multilingual speech has been researched by Dr Jean-Marc Dewaele and Adrian Furnham (2000). Studies done by M.W. Eysenck (1981) on personality and language had shown that extraverts benefited from having better short-term memories. He argued that anxious introverts can take longer to retrieve information stored in the brain, making their natural speech seem stilted. This effect is often referred to as *communicative anxiety*. This communicative anxiety is often observed in monolingual people learning a second language, where is it referred to as *foreign language anxiety*. The anxiety of getting it wrong or errors can inhibit a shy person from normal speech. Meanwhile, extroverts breeze through potentially stressful linguistic situations because they have more confidence and less fear of making mistakes. Dewaele and Furnham recorded conversations with 25 Flemish university students using French as their second language in a formal 'stressful' situation (a 10-minute oral exam) and an informal 'neutral' one (chatting about hobbies, studies or politics). In the informal situation they found that both extraverts and introverts had similar language skills. However, in the formal situation the introverts 'overloaded their working memory' and were less efficient at processing information. It follows that an extravert student may be better equipped to speak both languages than an introverted student, who is simply unable to 'find' the right words at the right time. The researchers concluded that the perceived stressfulness of the exam situation for introverts made them less fluent in French than they really were. Dewaele and Furnham described some of the students suffering from anxiety, commenting,

> This means their speech slows down, they hesitate more often, they tend to make more errors and they are unable to produce utterances of great length. (Dewaele & Furnham, 2000: 362)

In a recent online study, Dewaele *et al.* (2008) polled a wide range of 464 multilingual adults. The researchers asked participants about how anxious they felt using their second, third or fourth languages. Results showed that in a formal or classroom-based situation language anxiety was increased, and more relaxed informal extra-curricular language learning activities reduced stress levels.

In a secondary or high school setting, would introverted children have problems to retrieve linguistic information quickly enough too? This kind of pressure might lead to introverted children scoring less on oral tests in second-language studies. Salim Abu-Rabia (2004) observed 67 seventh-grade children in Israel studying English. He tested their level of achievement with written and reading tests and correlated the results with the student's levels of anxiety. Abu-Rabia found that student anxiety did lead to negative results, but the teachers had a role to play too. The teachers could off-set anxious students by making allowances for their verbal performance. These studies have been made on adolescents or young adults learning a second or third language. Do they also apply to children learning two or more languages? I asked the case-study families what they thought about extroversion and introversion with regard to their personal experiences with the question:

Do you think it helps to be an extrovert to excel in languages?

Eight of the 22 parents thought that being extrovert was an advantage because it would give a child more practice. Three mothers said that children who are shy or timid are often scared of making mistakes or sounding 'wrong', so they might prefer to not take the risk of using unfamiliar or new language. Alice, mother of two trilingual children, noted that her daughter is an outgoing child and is less worried about making grammatical mistakes and will keep talking even if her language is not always correct.

I think this is what is helping my older daughter, the fact that she is so outgoing! She isn't shy at all and just chatters away, in whatever language. What she says isn't necessarily grammatically correct, but at least she is chattering away to all and sundry.
Alice: German/Spanish/English in Austria (Lingua Franca) mother of Isabella (5) and Dominik (2)

Martine made the point that language is all about communication.

To speak a language means to communicate with the others. If you are an introvert, shy or timid you do not wish to communicate so much. So an extrovert person will be more appropriate to excel in languages.
Martine: French/English in Switzerland (OPOL) mother of mother of Tiéphaine (9) and Xavier (7)

Gerry remarked that being a more extrovert person encourages a more 'fearless' use of language, or trying out different ways of using language, a useful skill as children grow and must adapt their language to the wider world.

Introverted characteristics can limit one's learning and practice of a language. To learn a second language effectively, especially at an older age, it helps to be fearless and use the language widely and frequently. Shy or timid behaviour does not favour this necessity.
Gerry: English/Spanish in Canada (OPOL), mother of four children (aged 13, 11, 7 and 5)

On the other hand, other parents pointed out that being an extrovert was not the only skill needed in developing bilingualism Theresa, Claudia and Josie all noted that being an extrovert was perhaps not so important in the long run. Claudia remarks that being an extrovert is good for 'verbal exchanges' but children also need a good base in reading and writing skills. In these areas an introverted, or shy child, could shine.

For the verbal exchanges yes, being an extrovert is good, but not necessarily for comprehension or writing.
Claudia: Italian/Flemish/French/English multilingual family in France, mother of Milo (4) and Zeno (2)

I don't think it takes an extrovert to excel at languages although that probably helps to the extent that the extrovert will have more practice in a language. In my opinion, a keen interest in reading is far more important in language development.
Josie: Chinese/German/English trilingual family in Germany, mother of Niklas (12), Tobias (8) and Lukas (4)

As for being an extrovert, it probably helps, but it isn't necessary. I'm an introvert and people say my Spanish is near-native, but it probably would have been easier if I had been an extrovert. (Theresa: English/Spanish in Spain (OPOL), mother of Carmen (13), Rocio (11) and Violeta (9))

Martina and Christina thought that being an extrovert was simply not important.

I believe that being able to speak two or three languages gives you more confidence in yourself and makes you 'different' in a good way, in that you have something more than people who speak only one language.
Martina: Spanish/Italian/English trilingual family in Italy, mother of Alessia (8) and Gaia (6)

I know many extroverts with terrible language skills. I'd go as far as saying that introverts probably have an advantage when it comes to language learning.
Christina: English/German in Germany (OPOL), mother of Tom (15) and John (12)

The extrovert issue is a debated personality trait among the sample. It would seem likely that a child with an outgoing personality would benefit linguistically. The ability to 'chat' and engage others in conversation would help their development of vocabulary and accent, alongside learning how to adapt their speech to suit the interlocutor, or person they are talking to. This is especially valid in families where only one parent speaks the minority language. Having a child who is happy to talk to other speakers of a minority-language, for example, with friends of the parents, will increase the child's exposure and active use of the language. Being less concerned about making mistakes also helps language development in the early years when grammar and syntax are still emerging.

Children who are less outgoing or introvert do not necessarily lose out. Reserved or timid children may appreciate language learning through reading books or written creative work. In this situation children may feel more comfortable practicing languages in a smaller group or with someone they know well, like a grandparent or a family friend. A shy child may also benefit from practicing language with a sibling rather than with a stranger. The quieter children may also be listening in on conversations and picking up the grammatical rules, so when they feel ready they are confident enough to use the language. A quiet child, when presented with the right opportunity, might just start chatting away, surprising family and friends.

Perhaps language anxiety should be taken into account more when testing bilingual children? A formal school environment with emphasis on quick memory and verbal skills is not always suited to a more introverted child. In this case, parents might need to adapt language learning for introverted children through informal after-school or extracurricular activities. We should also bear in mind that some children have stages in their development when they are just not so talkative or chatty at home, like when they are starting school or going through adolescence and it should not worry parents too much.

A child's social skills could affect how they use languages. Being an *extrovert* can be an advantage, in formal situations like school and oral exams, but less outgoing children can do just as well too.

LANGUAGE FRICTION

His sister makes fun of the way he pronounces words …

One child is always correcting another one …

Our oldest child never lets the other child have his say!

- Not allowing the other sibling to talk.
- Laughing at sibling's wrong pronunciation or linguistic misunderstandings.
- Overcorrecting grammatical errors or phonological errors.

Inter-sibling conflict and rivalry are well-documented subjects in the literature for parents on child development. These inter-sibling wars are often referred to as *sibling rivalry* by child psychologists and family counselors. Birth order and gender are involved as first-, second- and last-born children juggle for attention. There can be hidden or open jealousy, competition, arguing, fighting or hostility to a new baby taking the parents' attention. According to psychologists Adele Faber and Elaine Mazlish (*Siblings Without Rivalry*, 2004) sibling rivalry is typically observed in half of all first-born children and is most intense between same-sex siblings who are close in age. Sibling rivalry can also be linked to the one or more of the children feeling that they are treated unfairly. It appears to be worse when the parents have 'inconsistent discipline practices', for example, when they punish one child harshly while letting another one get away with just a warning. Each sibling's personality, compatibility to share or ability to compromise can affect the level of sibling rivalry too.

In competing for parental attention, siblings can use language as a tool for usurping the other one. Common inter-sibling language tricks reported in case studies of both monolingual and bilingual families included not allowing other sibling to talk in one language, laughing at mistakes or overcorrecting grammatical errors. Older brothers and sisters can use overcomplicated or sophisticated language with a younger child, to confuse them or belittle them. The first-born child often has the upper hand in correcting siblings, sometimes playing the role of surrogate parent, but younger ones can be just as active in spotting mistakes or laughing at errors too. This language use is seen both at home and in the playground. At a certain level this inter-sibling language sparring can be a game; a safe way for siblings to learn from their linguistic mistakes, within the relatively safe family environment. However, if siblings become overzealous and communication becomes more negative in tone it can be upsetting and malicious. Professor Judy Dunn (*Sisters and Brothers*, 1985) noted the differing ways young siblings upset each other, with first-borns sometimes using language as a tool for attacking younger siblings. She says,

> During their early years, laterborn children are frequently more directly aggressive than their older siblings …. They may not be any more hostile-but they do express their aggression very directly and physically. Firstborns tend to be more **verbally** aggressive, criticizing and disparaging their younger brothers and sisters mercilessly. (Dunn, 1985: 71)

Siblings who are close in age may be competing to read, spell or write as well as their brother or sister, who is a few years ahead at school. This could lead to frustration and anger that the other one is always better. Even if it is a temporary stage it can cause concern to all those involved, especially to parents who have made efforts to encourage bilingualism. In a bilingual setting they can possibly lose confidence in speaking one language at home, sliding into passive language use over time or give up speaking one language permanently. This is a subject very much under-researched and there are few examples of this kind of language use in the literature on bilingualism.

However, one study by Victoria Obied (2009) observed four bilingual English/Portuguese families in Portugal, with children aged from eight to 17 years old. In one family there was conflict over the balance of language in the home. Nine-year-old Alexandre identified strongly with his father's Portuguese language and culture. Older brother, Marco, 13, was bilingual and tried to help his English mother encourage Alexandre to communicate more in English but, as Victoria observed,

> The mother and the older sibling attempt to scaffold Alexandre's English in the home, but Alexandre is often aggressive in his language use and he does not look to his older brother for help in literacy activities in the home: No, never! (Obied 2009: 710)

Victoria attributed the problem to the over-dominance of the Portuguese father's oral culture in the home, which was making it difficult for the English mother to transmit her culture through reading and writing. The older brother wanted to help out, but was rejected by his sibling and their communication had become negative and aggressive. In another English/Portuguese family, eight-year-old Claudia preferred to speak Portuguese at home with both parents and her six-year-old brother, Jorge. English had a minor role and Claudia encouraged her brother to speak Portuguese with her, thus limiting use of the minority language. Claudia appeared to not want her brother to become bilingual and blocked his chances to learn, either through her or with their mother. Victoria transcribed the conversation of the English mother offering to read a bedtime story in English. Claudia managed to divert the shared reading time into an argument, saying that she preferred the mother to read in Portuguese. In the end both children lost out on time with their mother reading in her first language.

Madalena Cruz-Ferreira (*Three's a Crowd: Acquiring Portuguese in a Trilingual Environment*, 2006), noted how her trilingual daughter, Karin, was captured on record employing pre-meditated strategies to undermine her siblings through games.

> One of {Karin's} favorite strategies was to invent complicated rules for a game of her own devising, painstakingly teach only a few of those rules to her siblings, and then start the game in such a way that it required immediate application of a rule that was known to her alone, dismissing her siblings bafflement on account of their lack of commonsense knowledge about game rules. (Cruz-Ferreira, 2006: 36)

Linguistic friction can also be linked to growing up and a teenager's need for independence and freedom. Stephen Caldas recounted a period of 'linguistic friction' at home, around the time their pre-adolescent son, John, aged 10, started fifth-grade at an English-language High School. Affected by his new peer group and school environment John spoke hardly any French, while his twin sisters, Valerie and Stephanie, were recorded as speaking 'more than 90%' French around the dinner table. This caused some friction in the home between the siblings, who had lost their sibling language of communication temporarily, as Stephen Caldas recounts:

> Our family language conflict grew increasingly violent. In January 1996, Valerie (8;8) was once so mad at John (10;8) for speaking English, that she threw a cushion at him, while screaming 'Parle français!!!' On another occasion a few weeks later, I heard the girls scream so violently at John to 'Parle français!!!' that I feared it would come to blows. (Caldas, 2006: 63)

John, understandably, retaliated to his sister's provocation, as recorded by his father,

> On one occasion I recorded John (age 10;8) firing back at Valerie, 'I have the right to speak any language I want to speak!' On several occasions John responded to Valerie's demands that he speak French by screaming back at her 'English! English! English!

The twins fought for a couple of years over which language was to be used between them, and then made an abrupt switch to English, when they were around age 10. Stephen Caldas remarked that at the time John's 'changed attitudes and speech' was not conducive to encouraging bilingual language skills. John's 'English only' stance probably contributed to the girls deciding to speak less French at home, even though they were still in bilingual schools and had plenty of exposure to French. It could be that the siblings decided that fighting over language use was futile. The case-study families had not experienced much language friction, but two mothers noted some tension in their children's language use. Brazilian mother, Lilian, commented that her older son sometimes forbids the younger one to speak in the majority language.

> *My oldest son provokes the youngest and one of the ways of taunting him is saying that he can speak English and the little one can't. My oldest son sometimes forbids his brother*

to speak English, because he says that he cannot really speak it. I think that if he were more accommodating in this sense his brother would develop even more in the foreign language. He flaunts his own fluency to his brother which I don't like.
Lilian: English/Portuguese in the United States (mL@H), mother of Kelvin (5) & Linton (3)

Another case-study mother, Gerry, says she has experienced:

Taunting due to accents or mispronunciations and teasing when errors occur by the older two boys toward the younger two children.
Gerry: English/Spanish in Canada (OPOL) mother of four children (aged 13, 11, 7 and 5)

In many families, language friction is short lived and linked to a particular event or incident. Siblings know each other well and have the means to use language to upset each other, regardless of parental intervention or disproval. In many cases it will work itself out as siblings find a common interest together, or begin to focus more on outside activities and friends. They need to learn to accept each other's personalities as they are and live together. However, in other families language friction may signal that children feel pressurized to change their language use at home to suit a bossy sibling, usually dropping the minority language. Parents may have to accept this sibling pressure or look for creative ways to encourage and reintroduce the language within the family.

Language *friction* is when the children use language to upset, annoy or insult each other. It can potentially lead to one language being under-used or dropped, but may be short lived.

SUMMARY

This chapter shows that siblings brought up in the same family can grow up to have very different language histories. Whether their genetic makeup, parental influence or peer pressure has the strongest influence remains debatable as researchers continue to investigate the effects of genes and the shared environment. Each child's unique mix of nature and nurture blends to make them react in certain ways to the world around them. Some children find learning languages easy while other children, even in the same family, struggle and are frustrated at their lack of fluency even after trying hard. Parents should be careful of having high expectations, and be aware that not all children love languages, in the same way that they might.

It appears that the children's personality or character can have an effect on the way they express themselves through language. Some children seem naturally attracted to communicating with people while other children find it hard to keep a conversation going. Extroverted or outgoing children may have an advantage in having more opportunity to practice language. They are less anxious about speaking in public or to strangers, and can score higher marks in oral tests. Quieter children use languages in different ways, possibly through reading and writing. However, in an informal situation a shy or timid child can feel comfortable using two or more languages.

Sibling rivalry can cause some language friction, at certain times, in the sibling's lives. One sibling starting school, becoming an adolescent or being in a different education system to another can cause a temporary breakdown in communication or negative use of language toward a sibling. These sibling differences are perhaps seen more clearly in a bilingual household, where parents are perhaps more tuned in to how their children speak or communicate than in monolingual families. This chapter highlights the fact that even with the best genetic inheritance, parental support and encouragement of languages in the home, there's no guarantee that all the children will turn out bilingual. In Chapter 8 we will look at some special cases in terms of family bilingualism; twins, adopted children and step-families.

Further reading on individual differences

Abu-Rabia, S. (2004) Teachers' role, learners' gender differences, and FL anxiety among seventh-grade students studying English as a FL. *Educational Psychology* 24 (5), 711–21.

Caldas, S.J. (2006) *Raising Bilingual-Biliterate Children in Monolingual Cultures*. Clevedon: Multilingual Matters.

Chomsky, N. (1968) *Language and Mind*. New York: Harcourt Brace and World Inc.

Cruz-Ferreira, M. (2006) *Three's a Crowd: Acquiring Portuguese in a Trilingual Environment*. Clevedon: Multilingual Matters.

Dewaele, J.M. and Furnham, A. (2000) Personality and speech production: A pilot study of second language learners. *Personality and Individual Differences* 28, 355–365.

Dewaele, J.M., Petrides, K.V. and Furnham, A. (2008) The effects of trait emotional intelligence and sociobiographical variable on communicative anxiety and foreign language anxiety among adult multilinguals: A review and empirical investigation. *Language Learning* 58 (4).

Dodd, B., Hemsley, G. and Stow, C. (2008) Bilingualism and learning difficulties: Separating fact from fiction. *The Bilingual Family Newsletter* 25 (2), 5–6.

Dunn, J. and Plomin, R. (1990) *Separate Lives: Why Siblings Are So Different*. New York: Basic Books.

Eysenck, M.W. (1981) Learning, memory and personality. In H.J. Eysenck (ed.) *A Model for Personality*. Berlin: Springer-Verlag.

Faber, A. and Mazlish, E. (2004) *Siblings without Rivalry*. London: Piccadilly.

Fantini, A.E. (1985) *Language Acquisition of a Bilingual Child*. Clevedon: Multilingual Matters.

Harris, J.R. (1998) *The Nurture Assumption*. New York: W.W. Norton & Co.

Huss, L. (2003) Creating a bilingual family in a monolingual country. *The Bilingual Family Newsletter* 20 (3), 4–7.

King, K. and Mackay, A. (2007) *The Bilingual Edge: Why, When and How to Teach Your Child a Second Language*. New York: HarperCollins.

Laversuch, I.M. (2006) Stuttering and bilingualism: Finding the courage to be heard. *The Bilingual Family Newsletter* 23 (2), 6–7.

Lerner, J.V., Nitz, K., Talwar, R. and Lerner, R.M. (1989) On the functional significance of temperamental individuality: A developmental contextual view of the concept of goodness of fit.' In G.A. Kohnstamm, J.E. Bates and M.K. Rothbart (eds) *Temperament in Childhood*. Chichester: John Wiley.

Obied, V. (2009) How do siblings shape the language environment in bilingual families? *International Journal of Bilingual Education and Bilingualism* 12 (6), 705–720.

Pinker, S. (2002) *The Blank Slate*. New York: Allen Lane.

Plomin, R. (1990) *Nature and Nurture: An Introduction to Human Behavioral Genetics*. CA: Brooks/Cole.

Sulloway, J.F. (1997) *Born to Rebel: Birth Order, Family Dynamics and Creative Lives*. New York: Vintage Books

Thomas, A., Chess, S. and Birch, H. (1968) *Temperament and Behavior Disorders in Children*. New York: New York University Press.

Valenzuela, M. (2004) Family language strategies on the move: A balancing act. *The Bilingual Family Newsletter* 21 (4), 7.

Youngblade, L.M. and Dunn, J. (1995) Individual differences in young children's pretend play with mother and sibling: Links to relationships and understanding of other people's feelings and beliefs. *Child Development* 66 (5), 1472–1492.

Note: You can read more about the families of Theresa, Alice, Martina, Odile, Martine, Gerry, Claudia, Josie, Christina and Lilian in *Family Profiles* at the end of the book.

Chapter 8

Bilingualism and Twins, Adoption, Single Parents and Step-Families

This chapter looks at families from a different perspective – twins, adopted children, single parent families and children with half-brothers and sisters. How do these special families deal with bilingualism? Do bilingual twins speak the same languages or is there a personal preference for one language? We consider the language behaviors of twins in relation to case studies. With adopted children there are sensitive issues relating to the child's heritage or native language within their new family. Should parents support their adopted child's first language at home or concentrate on developing the language of their new home?

Separation, divorce and bereavement can affect bilingual families. How do single parents maintain bilingualism on their own? Is it possible for one parent to support two languages single-handedly? What happens if the single parent decided to remarry? This leads to the next issue – step-families. Step-families, or blended families, need to find a way to communicate through one language, while still retaining parental languages too. Step-families, with two or more existing family languages or a new family language, may have to find a 'common' language for daily communication.

TWINS AND LANGUAGE USE

Our twins talked a little later than children their own age, but once they were talking there was no stopping them

On average there are 3.5 sets of identical twins in every 1000 births. Monozygotic twins are identical and result from the splitting of one egg during fertilization. Identical twins have a genetic similarity of 100%. Fraternal or dizygotic twins are formed from two separate eggs being fertilized at the same time. According to Robert Plomin, a behavioral geneticist, fraternal twins are no more alike than ordinary siblings and share only 50% of their genes. Fraternal twins can be different in size, physical attributes or personalities. Judith Rich Harris (*No Two Alike Human: Nature and Human Individuality*, 2006) investigated the theory that identical twins sharing the same genes, environment and lifestyle would have the same personality characteristics. Judith found that sets of twins, even twins cojoined by the head or body, can have different personalities. Even with a common genetic background and a shared home there was still an unexplained difference, as Judith says,

> Identical twins have different social experiences because the members of their community see them as unique individuals ... people who know them pick up on these little differences and use them to distinguish the twins. (Harris, 2006: 247)

Judith argued that each twin can react differently to various relationships in their world. One twin might become more interested in certain areas, such as school or a sport, or want to achieve different goals to their twin. Close family of twins and friends of twins are usually able to tell twins apart too, from small (or wide) differences in their behavior or physical appearance. Parents might find one child slightly stronger or weaker, quieter or chatty, one might prefer sugary snacks and the other salty food. This difference in character was highlighted by Tessa Livingstone in the British television program and accompanying book (*Child of Our Time*, 2005) which has followed 25 children since their birth in 2000. The sample included a set of girl triplets, Mabel, Alice and Phoebe (who also have three older siblings). In the book, which accompanied the series, the triplets were nearly five, and Tessa observed,

> Mabel, Alice and Phoebe have had different temperaments since they were born. As toddlers, Mabel was the tomboy and wanted lots of hugs; Alice was the dominant one – the princess of the family – and Phoebe was quiet and mischievous. By the time they were three the children had their own language. (Livingstone, 2005: 18)

The researchers remarked that Phoebe had a mild speech impediment, around age three, but by the time she was four she had caught up and was talking properly.

Language disorders are often common in twins or multiple births. Australian speech therapist, Caroline Bowen, in an online article on twins informed parents;

> Late onset of speech, and speech and language difficulties, including stuttering, are more common in twins than in singletons. This is because twins are frequently premature or low birth weight babies, and their parents may have less time to attend to them individually and to help them develop verbal skills.

Several studies over the last 20 years have suggested that twins, on average, are more prone to language delay. In a study done on young preschool twins Tomosello, Mannle and Kruger (1986) concluded that the parents of young twins simply had less time to talk to each twin individually. The reduced language input, could lead to delayed speech. There may be more of an inclination for parents to let the children talk to each other, since they are natural play companions who spend most of their day together. Another factor is the physical nature of many twins, who are often born prematurely or are below normal birth weight, and can be about six months behind in language development.

TEDS (see box) is a longitudinal research project which aims to find out more about twins. This UK/USA collaborative project allows researchers from various fields to follow the development of young twins. More than 15,000 pairs of twins were enrolled in TEDS. The twins were assessed at age two, three, four and seven years of age, to investigate genetic and environmental contributions to change and continuity in language and cognitive development.

One branch of the TEDS project focuses on communication disorders, mild mental impairment and behavior problems. A team (Philip Dale *et al.*, 1998) looked specifically at the 5% of

---

The *Twins Early Development Study* (TEDS)

Robert Plomin (Institute of Psychiatry in London, UK)

Philip Dale (University of Washington, USA)

15,000 twins born in UK from 1994 to 1996
Tested at age 2, 4 and 7 years of age.

For an overview of project,
see Trouton *et al.* (2002)

---

the sample who had early language delay. They tracked around 3000 sets of two-year-old twins from the TEDS study (1044 identical, 1006 same-sex and 989 opposite-sex twins). In general, both identical and fraternal twins scored very similarly in vocabulary tests. However, the brother or sister of an identical twin with a language delay had 81% chance of having the same problem. A fraternal twin had only a 42% chance of having the same language issue. The team concluded that language delay was a genetic factor, and that the environment and parental input made little difference. In a later testing of the twins at age four (Viding *et al.*, 2004) the team replicated the study, and concluded that genes do have a 'strong influence' on twins who have severe language impairment. Nevertheless, there was hope for some of the twins, as Dale comments,

> We know from longitudinal studies that many children with language delays at two years do prove to be 'late bloomers' who subsequently catch up with their peers.

Twinslist, an online research and information website run by the University of Southern California reported a number of young twins communicating through non-verbal gestures and having limited vocabulary. Twins appear to have a special intuitive understanding for each other, which cannot be compared to ordinary siblings. David Crystal (*The Cambridge Encyclopedia of Language*, 1987) comments,

> Observers have been struck by the intuitive way in which one twin is able to respond very rapidly to what the other has just said, and how the first twin is able to anticipate when to stop. They very seldom talk at the same time … They know each other's rhythms, and each is able to predict a great deal of what the other is likely to say. (Crystal, 1987: 247)

Twins can sometimes even create their own private language, known as an *idiglossia*. Crystal estimates that as many as 40% of twins develop some form of this 'private-speech', especially around their second year. Mieke Schuller (2002) reviewed the research done on twin language and explained,

> The most drastic form in which twin language development can culminate is the development of a private language, which is hard to understand for any person other than the twins. (Schuller, 2002: 3)

This twin-language can be an immature version of their home language or it can have a unique vocabulary or grammar, invented by the twins. Schuller noted that twin language does not often last beyond childhood. Most parents dismiss it in the early years as 'baby-talk', and only become concerned if it goes on into the fourth or fifth year. By the time the twins start preschool or primary school most of their speech delay is a thing of the past, although some retain articulation problems. This puts forward the view that twins do not talk much because they don't need to. It is perhaps not until they are in an unfamiliar school environment and need to socialize more with their peer group that they are forced to speak more. On a positive note, a Danish study published in the British Medical Journal (Christensen *et al.*, 2006) tested twins at age 15 and 16, and found very little difference in IQ levels. They concluded this was due to improved early pediatric support for twins born prematurely, who previously suffered from brain damage.

BILINGUAL TWINS

There are very few academic studies on bilingual twins. This could be because researchers cannot always accurately identify the twin's speech independently. The twins can sound exactly the same, with identical speech patterns, intonation or accents. When typed up it can be hard to see much difference between the speech of 'Twin A' and 'Twin B'. Therefore, taped or recorded speech is often combined and rated as if it were one child. One of the most extensive and cohesive reports of life with two languages and twins was compiled by Stephen Caldas on the language use of his identical twin daughters, Valerie and Stephanie. At times, Caldas had problems to identify which twin was speaking in his taped recording of family mealtimes, and was sometimes obliged to rate the twins collectively for purposes of data analysis. Nevertheless, he gave many examples of each daughter's speech, and their evolving individual attitudes to each language. In the early years, Caldas was concerned that the twins were rather slow in starting to speak, and commented,

> ... our twins had in essence two strikes against them: they had two languages to sort out and learn while being part of a twinship which researchers note inhibits speech. (Caldas, 2006: 47)

After a late start, the girls began to speak at age two, using one and two-word sentences, and imitating their four-year-old brother, John. By age three the twins were speaking 'normally' (confirmed by a screening by a speech pathologist) and by age five were scoring high on school 'readiness' tests. Would the girls achieve the same academic scores? Not necessarily. Caldas collected data regularly from his daughter's teachers and tested his three children's French proficiency up until they were teenagers.

In a test administered (see chart below) when the twins were in 5th Grade (around age eleven) both girls had a similar average – Valerie 40.6 and Stephanie 40.5 (out of 50). The twins were also asked to self-report their level of their French skills at age 10 and 15. Here the girls differed. In the first test Valerie gave herself 43, while Stephanie rated herself at 36. Five years later, when the twins were retested, Valerie selected 41, and her sister 37. To put this into context, their older brother, John, scored 36.6 on average in school tests and self-reported 31 and 41 respectively. At age 15, Valerie and John appear to have more in common, but the two girls have very close academic scores. However, looking at their scores over time shows that sometimes Valerie excelled, and at other times it was Stephanie. They did not always follow the same

French Proficiency Tests (out of 50)			
	John	*Valerie*	*Stephanie*
Teachers Average	36.6	40.6	40.5
Self report 1	31	43	36
Self report 2	41	41	37

pattern, and each girl had her particular highs and lows in terms of French proficiency. We might have expected the girls to follow the same learning pattern and have the same attitude to French as each other. Caldas wrote,

> Perhaps these findings taken together suggest that the children's evolving French proficiency (or their perceptions of this proficiency) differ in meaningful ways – even for twins who share the same genotypes and linguistic environments. Could the children's differing competences on individual measures of their French proficiency simply reflect the differences in their own unique personalities? (Caldas, 2006: 185)

This subtle difference in language use and preference was mirrored in other parents' descriptions of their twins individual language use. For example, in Family #95, an English/Spanish family living in Mexico with their three-year-old twin girls, the mother observed that one girl is 'more verbal and the other more physical' than her sister. This did not affect their fluency or language preferences though. In another family, there was a more marked difference. Family #16, a Spanish/English family with a Venezuelan mother and English father, lives in the United Kingdom. Their twin boys, age four, speak English fluently (their strongest language) and they use English together. The mother noted that twin A speaks Spanish at an 'intermediate' level while twin B is at 'beginner' level. Interestingly, twin A prefers to speak to his mother in Spanish, while twin B prefers English. The mother comments that both children have refused to speak Spanish, but often mix languages and add Spanish words to their English at home.

The Twinslist online website and forum has a special section for bilingual parents. Here is an excerpt from a mother talking about her English/Hebrew bilingual fraternal twins:

> *Our son is much more verbal, and uses mainly English. Our daughter uses more Hebrew words, but she has a smaller active vocabulary. When they were beginning to talk with each other it was mostly in English (before they would communicate with glances, gestures, etc.). At that age they did not communicate much verbally with each other at daycare. Now they speak Hebrew between themselves in daycare, and a mix at home.*

In my survey of 105 families there were five sets of twins. Family #78 is a French family living in the United Kingdom, with bilingual parents. They have fraternal twins; a boy and a girl who are seven years old. These twins are very similar linguistically, both speaking French fluently and English at an intermediate level. The family has lived in England for less than three years and French remains strong in the home environment. The twins have the same language preferences when they read, watch television or talk to their parents. When talking together the mother notes that they 'very often mix both languages in one single sentence.' This was echoed in an English/French family living in France with a seven-year-old daughter and three-year-old boy twins. The mother comments:

> *I've noticed that our older child talks to the twins in the language of the adult who is with them. She is fully bilingual. The twins speak a mixture of French and English back to her and together, with more French than English. They have their own way of making up words that their sister sometimes does not understand!*

Another parent mentioned that her twin Italian/English girls,

> *... talk for each other and explain what the other means. They often communicate in a nonverbal way and don't always need to talk to each other to understand what they mean. The girls have the same overall language preferences at home, but we think that one child is slightly more 'verbal' than the other.*

There were two case study families who had twins – Irene and Lisa. Irene has two boys, aged five, who speak French and Korean. Both mothers commented on their twin's shared language use and the complicity they share, saying, 'They seem to usually know what the other wants to do without speech.' Lisa has two 14-year girl English/Hebrew speaking twins and has watched their language development over the years. Lisa reports,

> *Rachel and Sarah were involved in an academic language study until they were 36 months. Both had some degree of delay until around 14–16 months. After that, both were above average (75th and 60th percentile)*

Now her daughters are in the 8th grade and are fluently bilingual, Lisa finds her daughters' characters affect their slightly different ways of expressing themselves:

> *At this point, their language skills are pretty similar. Rachel, who is more outgoing, is more likely to slip into slang "Ya know, like," in both languages. Sarah tends to be more precise; she's very aware of grammatical rules and correct usage.*

These comments on twins are just a brief snapshot of language use in the family. It would be necessary to test the individual language use and perception of bilinguality of each twin in a long-term study before reaching any solid conclusions. However, it can be said that twins, in general, do appear to have a similar preference for languages, although one twin can be more or less talkative or interested in languages. Twins can help each other out, and may benefit from a shared non-linguistic understanding. There may be less need to talk in their relationship, which could mean a possible delay in speech in the early years but this can be overcome when they do begin to talk. The choice of languages as their shared language is an important factor. The risk is that they could jointly decide *not* to speak one language, an issue that might be harder to resolve than with ordinary siblings who have different peer groups.

> Bilingual *twins* may have some early language delay. They can have similar or differing language preferences or abilities.

ADOPTION AND BILINGUALISM

We wanted to show our new daughter that we care about her past and hope that if we speak a little of her language it might help her settle in.

There is very little research available on international adoptions involving a child speaking a different language to the home he or she is adopted into. There is even less information on children adopted into bilingual homes and whether they become bilingual. What we do know is that, in general, adopted children lose their first language, or mother tongue. The majority or country language takes over within just a few years and the first language fades away over time. Age of the child is an important factor. Since the majority of adoptions are babies or young children their first language may not be developed or active when they are adopted. Older children, over the age of three or four may well have an established first language, which needs to be taken into consideration in the early days. Parents might have a period when their child is speaking a different language to them in their home. Some parents may consider speaking the adopted child's mother tongue or first language.

Iman Makeba Laversuch (*The Bilingual Family Newsletter*, 2004a) wrote an excellent article for parents about the issue of adopting a child and preserving their first language. She observed that:

> In the not so distant past, parents who adopted children from abroad were encouraged to break all ties with their child's country of origin. (Laversuch, 2004a: 6)

Consequently, these children grew up with a feeling they were missing something. Some of these adopted children found themselves drawn toward learning their first language, or mother tongue, in later life. Other older children or adults felt frustrated by their inability to speak their first language or mother tongue. This could result in what Iman describes as:

> … a double rootlessness: estranged from the country they were raised in and alienated from the country they were born in. (Laversuch, 2004a: 6)

Iman reports that things are changing now and parents are now keen to learn about their adopted child's culture and, in some cases, their first language. This embracing of the adopted child's culture can be positive and help the whole family adjust to a new life. The issue of well-meaning adoptive parents speaking the heritage language is not always so simple though. Hearing their mother tongue can provoke a negative reaction in the child so Iman urges parents to discuss with professionals before embarking on a first-language/culture immersion, warning,

> In some case the use of first language may dredge up memories of separation, neglect and abuse. (Laversuch, 2004a: 6)

The practical question 'What do parents do when they want to adopt a child, but do not speak the child's first language?' was discussed by Colin Baker (*A Parents' and Teachers' Guide to Bilingualism*, 2007). Colin advised parents to consider supporting the heritage language as a way to bring a sense of belonging and increase self-esteem for the adopted child. To prepare for the arrival of the child the parents-to-be can learn some of the first language initially; a few simple phrases, greetings and child-specific vocabulary. Parents can scaffold this with extra input from other people who speak the child's language. Materials such as books, videos, internet and satellite television in the child's native language can play a part too. Colin also advises a careful choice of school, where the child will feel accepted as a bicultural bilingual,

> What adopting parents can do is to provide their children with a wider set of choices with respect to languages and cultures. To give an adopted child the chance of retaining your language, of a bicultural or multicultural heritage, is to give freedom and power to the child. The parent who insists on ignoring and burying the child's linguistic and cultural origins can so easily be restricting and constraining the child. (Baker, 2007: 27)

Even if the parents are committed to providing support for another culture or language, and the child accepts the intercultural involvement, the siblings are not always so keen. T. Berry Brazelton and Joshua Sparrow (*Understanding Sibling Rivalry: The Brazelton Way*, 2005) discuss 'Cross-Racial and Cross-Cultural' adoptions, from an American perspective. They noted the potential strong feelings of identity that can arise between siblings when a child is adopted from another country or culture. Brazelton and Sparrow comment,

> At 4 and 5 years, children become curious about differences. At this age, they don't understand what they might mean to others. As they wonder, they're likely to blurt out: 'You look different. You're not even from America'. (Brazelton & Sparrow, 2005: 74)

Brazelton and Sparrow advised parents to find older children and adults from the adopted child's race or culture 'whom he can admire'. This could help the adopted child answer questions of identity and culture which might be troubling him or her. The decision to support an adopted child's first language does depend on the age of the child, and whether he or she speaks the first language. The agreement of the parents and other siblings to work at supporting another language in the home is important too. First or heritage language use can benefit a child but only with the implicit understanding that the adopted child may prefer *not* to speak his or her first language too, which should be respected.

INTERNATIONAL ADOPTIONS

Each case of international adoption is unique in the combination of parental, country and adopted child language. Actress and celebrity, Angelina Jolie, is well known for her high-profile international adoptions. She is a mother of six children; three adopted (from three different countries) and three biological children with actor Brad Pitt. The family lives in America and the language of the family is English. Angelina's mother was French-Canadian and Angelina has been recorded as saying that she wants to bring up her children with French as their second language. Angelina first adopted a Cambodian baby boy, Maddox Chivan, in 2001 when he was seven months old. Four years later, in 2005, she adopted a six-month-old girl, Zahara Marley, from Ethiopia. Her new partner, Brad Pitt, became the step-father of Maddox and Zahara, in 2006. Their first biological child, daughter Shiloh Nouvel, was born the same year in Namibia, Africa. In 2007 the couple adopted a Vietnamese boy, Pax Thien, who was three and half years old. Their biological twins Knox Léon and Vivienne Marcheline, a girl and a boy, were born a year later, in France. Angelina is reported to employ teachers who teach Cambodian and Vietnamese to Maddox and Pax, and the parents encourage the music and culture of each adopted child's heritage.

There was an interesting query in *The Bilingual Family Newsletter* (2004) from a couple regarding adoption. Roger Horney, a British man, and his Singaporean wife, who spoke English, Cantonese and some Mandarin, had adopted a 19-month-old girl, Sasha, from China. Sasha was having some difficulty with her new language, English. The parents wanted to know how they could help their daughter acquire English 'as naturally as possible'. Roger explained that the situation was complicated by the Chinese dialects, saying:

> It is very difficult to know what Chinese 'dialects' Sasha has been exposed to, let alone which language is, literally, her mother tongue. Almost certainly she had heard Mandarin but may also have heard the Hunan dialect local to the orphanage. Given all this, my wife decided not to speak Cantonese to Sasha or, at this stage, Mandarin. We are concentrating completely on English.

The reply was that in the short-term Roger and his wife should make English a priority to prepare Sasha for future schooling in English. Chinese could come later, through organized language classes. The family had close links with the Chinese-speaking community in Singapore, and with other families in the United Kingdom who had adopted Chinese babies, who could support them.

Six months later, another bilingual family responded to Roger's letter, giving their story on siblings, adoption and bilingualism (*The Bilingual Family Newsletter*, 2003). Tracey Martin, an English-speaker, lived in Thailand with her Thai husband and their adopted son, Ben. Both parents were bilingual, in English and Thai, and followed the

OPOL approach with Ben. They fostered a second son, Bin, from Thailand. To help him adjust Tracey describes how she translated for him in the early days,

> I wanted him to learn English so he could feel fully part of this bilingual family but I also wanted him to feel at home and understand what was going on. I therefore adopted the strategy of saying things to him in English and then repeating them in Thai and vice versa.

This continued until Bin felt comfortable using English with Tracey. She described the transition as 'painless and quick', due to an English-language summer school which Bin attended, and his determination to be 'part of the family.' The family now lives in The Gambia and Bin attends an English-language school. Although we don't know the ages of the two boys it appears that they are close in age and formed a bond through their shared common language (Thai). Bin is able to support his first language, even though he lives away from Thailand, because he still speaks to his brother, Ben, in Thai.

Barbara Zuer-Pearson (*Raising a Bilingual Child*, 2008) included a case study on an adopted child and her mother who followed a *non-native* language strategy. The parents are both Americans and the mother, Rosemary, learnt Spanish as a 'late learner'. They wanted to preserve their daughter's Latina identity and give her the chance to speak to people from her birth country. Barbara reported that Rosemary has spoken exclusively to her daughter, Caridad, in Spanish, '… from the day she met her in Guatemala when Cari was ten months old'. Rosemary was initially worried she would not have enough vocabulary to keep up with Carida's developing speech. Spanish-speaking friends and other families who had adopted children who spoke Spanish as a first language supported her efforts. The strategy paid off as Barbara reports that although Cari 'rarely' replies to her mother in Spanish, she understands and can communicate well with Spanish-speaking people. Cari is now 13 years old, and has a common bond between mother and daughter, as Barbara describes:

> Cari and her mom share an interest in Latin music and swap songs all the time, more and more as Cari gets older and knows a wider range of music than her mother. Overall, Rosemary says it has been easier than she thought. She never thought she'd be able to continue it for so long. (Zuer-Pearson, 2008: 184)

Violeta Garcia-Mendoza wrote an article on her international adoption of three young children in the *Multilingual Living* online magazine. Originally from a Spanish/English bilingual family herself Violeta married an American and the couple chose to adopt from Guatemala because of Violeta's link with the Spanish language. They adopted two children initially, Maya and Joaquin, and then the sister of Joaquin joined the family soon after. At home Violeta speaks Spanish and her husband English, as she explains,

> In practice, because I feel Spanish and English are both important to my identity, we chose not to employ a strict one parent-one language strategy, opting instead

for a more flexible approach. My husband speaks more English with our children than Spanish, which he's learning increasingly by being surrounded; I speak more Spanish than English at home. Because we both work from home, our kids do end up hearing about the same of each language. (Garcia-Mendoza, 2008: 29)

Violeta recommends finding other families with similar international adoptions or people from the adoptive country to give cultural support to the minority language. These five families, each with its own unique mélange of language and cultures, have all helped to make the transition for the child from orphanage or birth family to their home as smooth as possible.

> Families who *adopt* children may need to consider how or whether they will support the child's *first* or *heritage* language.

SINGLE PARENTS

I'm speaking my ex-husband's language at home these days, or I fear that my children will simply forget it and one day they might regret not being able to speak it.

In terms of bilingual families case studies rarely discuss one-parent families, even though there are single parents all around the world who are raising their children bilingually, by choice or through a change of circumstances. In my first book (*Language Strategies for Bilingual Families*, 2004) I interviewed two single mothers who were raising their children with two languages. Both mothers were keen to keep the father's language active in the child's life. However, this is not always the case, often when bilingual parents split up one parent goes back to their home country and a child has significantly less contact with one parent and their language. This sudden move from a bilingual to monolingual home can be traumatic and confusing for children as Iman Makeba Laversuch (*The Bilingual Family Newsletter*, 2004b) perceptively writes,

> Before divorce, many families freely switch languages. After a divorce, these homes may be split into two separate monolingual households, each with their separate agendas. When this happens, children may begin to feel (or be made to feel) that speaking the language of the one of their parents will automatically be perceived as disloyalty to their other parent. (Laversuch, 2004b: 2–3)

Iman recommends that parents need to renegotiate a family language policy to keep communication open between parents and children and try to avoid negative connotations against the language of the partner who has left the family home. Some children move homes and find themselves immersed in a new culture with a language they only spoke with a few people before. Barbara Zuer-Pearson (*Raising a Bilingual Child*, 2008) profiled Carmen, a young girl from a bilingual family whose parents had divorced. Carmen moved from mainly monolingual New England to her mother's native country, Puerto Rica, when she was 10 years old. Carmen spent four years with her mother, before returning to complete high school in New England with her father. Although she initially had a hard time adapting to school in Spanish Carmen benefited from her experience in the long-term. Carman, now a young adult, commutes between her two countries and has a job where she uses both languages on a daily basis. Barbara noted that Carmen had,

> ... much better command of Spanish than that of her younger brothers, who stayed in the US with their father, except for summer vacations in Puerto Rica. (Zuer-Pearson, 2008: 191)

Colin Baker (*The Parents' and Teachers' Guide to Bilingualism*, 2007) recommends that the extended family is involved, with the support of aunts, uncles, neighbors and friends, to give children enough exposure to both languages. As he says,

> It is possible to raise a child bilingually inside a one-parent family. This is simply because a child's bilingualism may be acquired outside the mother-child or father-child relationship. (Baker, 2007: 14)

Single parents who are bilingual can choose to speak the other parent's language to the child at home, following a *non-native* strategy, or a mix of both languages. Some parents chose to support the other parental language through schooling in the minority language or an external *time & place* strategy. Barbara Zuer-Pearson reported on an American single mother, Shelley, who employed extra help from the community she lived in to help maintain her ex-husband's language, Chinese. Shelley's ex-husband was from Taiwan and they had two children, Mark, 14 and Susan, 8 (adopted at age 11 months from China). Shelley wanted to keep their Chinese heritage language active and experienced varying degrees of success with a part-time Chinese nanny and Saturday schools. She finally found a dual-language primary school program which proved to be the best solution, and hired extra Chinese tutors to practice conversation after-school. Mark is described as 'doing well' and has some Chinese friends (who are bilingual) but is limited in his motivation to speak Chinese. Susan joined the school in the kindergarten year, and was described as enjoying learning in Chinese. Shelley had made a lot of effort to find the right way to include Chinese in their family but accepted that in the long-run her children need to make the effort too. In that respect she is stepping back and letting the children make the initiative to learn their father's language. Barbara observed the family, saying,

> ... it seems to his mother ... that her efforts have not given him {Mark} a useful command of the second language (Chinese) ... Shelley is resigned to the idea that the next language-learning efforts will have to come from Mark. (Zuer-Pearson, 2008: 207)

Victoria Obied (2002) conducted a study on four English/Portuguese families in Portugal and their literacy skills. One set of siblings were part of single-parent family. Martin, 11, Janet, 16 and Justin, 17, live with their Scottish mother. Their father was a multilingual Croatian who spoke five languages. The father spoke a mix of Portuguese and English with his children and never spoke Croatian. The parents separated when Martin was two years old. Victoria observed that each child had had a different language history. Justin had a clear split of English at home/Portuguese outside the home. Janet had English at home too, but preferred to play with her brother in Portuguese at home. Martin had less family contact and more exposure to the community language,

> Martin's early language experience contrasted with his two older siblings as the parents divorced and the mother became a single parent. Martin had more contact with Portuguese neighbors in the community and a Portuguese babysitter. (Obied, 2002: 716)

The mother mixed languages regularly, a strategy which suited her and the children. She worked full-time and had limited time to support the children's language skills. The mother's challenge was how to keep English active with her three children, who were old enough to make their own decisions on language use at home. On a positive note, Martin was keen to learn English from his mother. Single parents can, and do, maintain two languages in the house, but what happens when a parent re-marries or starts another relationship?

Single parents need to consider how they can maintain the other parental language, via the extended family, schooling or the siblings.

SIBLINGS WITH HALF-SISTERS AND BROTHERS

> *When we moved in with my new partner we had to decide which language was the 'family' one, so no-one could say they were left out. But I still speak 'my' language one-to-one with my kids.*

What happens when two families blend to create another family? The new stepfather or stepmother might have their own children, from previous marriages or relationships, who come to live with them. The new couple might also decide to have another baby together. In bilingual families one parent may feel that they need to rewrite the family language strategy, with the arrival of a new step-father or step-mother. In a family where the new step-parent does not understand one language this might be a necessary step for communication, although parents can still speak directly to their children in their first language. Another issue for children in bilingual families is the risk it that one parental language can be sidelined or potentially lost if contact is reduced with that parent. Practical problems of organizing children to spend time with both parents can be complicated by parents who have moved back to their home country, or now live in another country. When a new family is formed a minority-language can be at risk. Finnish/English bilingual Nina Majakari (*The Bilingual Family*

Newsletter, 2006) traced her roots with two cultures and identities. Nina's father was Finnish and fluent in English after living in England for many years. Nina's parents had met when her step-brother was eight years old, and she was born three years later. Sadly, the father felt he would never return to Finland, and that Finnish was a 'useless' language so when his daughter was born in 1978 he chose not to speak Finnish with her. He thought that it was more 'beneficial' for his daughter to have a 'good command' of English. In the northern English town, where the family lived 30 years ago, speaking a 'foreign' language in public might have been frowned on. Nina explains that her parents were concerned for her older step-brother,

> I was born when he was 11, therefore there was a risk that speaking Finnish with me could have alienated him. Evidently, complexity exists within bilingual and multilingual families. (Majakari, 2006: 6)

Her father tried to teach Nina Finnish when she was four, but the idea 'died a natural death.' The family did engage in some cultural traditions, such as a Finnish Christmas (opening their presents on Christmas Eve) or a celebrating a Finnish springtime festival. But her father felt uncomfortable using 'his' language with his close family. In fact, he acknowledged in the article that he now realized Nina had missed out having contact with her extended family in Finland. It was Nina herself who instigated Finnish, inspired by a visit to extended family in Finland when she was 11. She went on to study Finnish as a student and eventually moved to live in Helsinki when she was an adult.

One family who completed the online survey, Family #97, had a trio of languages at home (Dutch, Russian and English) and six half-sisters and brothers (due to the limited nature of the online study it is not possible to know if the children all live together or spend some time with their respective mothers or fathers). The father was British and currently married to a Russian woman. They lived in the Netherlands and spoke English together. The mother spoke Russian and the father a mix of English and Dutch. Two of the children were Russian-born (his current wife's children) – Child 1 was born in 1983 and Child 3 in 1995. The family also included the three children of the first wife, a Dutch-speaker – Child 2 (born in 1992), Child 4 (also born in 1995) and Child 5 (no date of birth available) who were all born in the Netherlands. The couple also has a joint sixth child, born in the Netherlands. In this family there was a real need for a 'common' language, to bring together the two Russian-speaking siblings, the three Dutch-speaking siblings and the new baby. In the end, Russian lost out and became the minority-language. Only Child 1, a girl, continues to speak Russian, the others all list Dutch/English as their equal first or strongest languages. Child 1 still speaks Russian to her mother; despite the fact that the others prefer English. The older children attend Dutch-language schools, with Child 1 and 4 having some English support at school too. Between the siblings a mix of English and Dutch is the preferred choice. Child 1 speaks some Russian to her siblings (but they reply to her in another language) and still reads and watches television in Russian, while the others prefer English as their language of reading and television. The father states that his sixth child is becoming trilingual, which is bringing Russian back into family use. However, Russian remains the endangered language since the siblings do not feel comfortable using it together in front of their Dutch step-siblings.

As we can see in these brief snapshots of step-siblings there is a need for a common language, between new siblings and their stepfather or stepmother. But it is also important to not 'lose' one language in the rush to set up a new family. In an ideal world each language would have equal weight, but unfortunately languages can be pushed out by a dominant majority country language. Parents living away from their country need to consider carefully their options for schooling or extra lessons in the minority language, and try to organize cultural trips and visits to their home country.

> Parents in bilingual families with *stepchildren* need to consider the language of family communication, without losing contact with their own children's language.

SUMMARY

This chapter shows some of the challenges of bilingual families; twins, adoption, single-parenting and step-families. All of these issues may need some measured thought on the part of the parents as to how they encourage language use, maintain heritage or minority languages and create a family home which welcomes children from orphanages or other families. Families in all of these situations need to carefully consider the language of the school the children attend, which can affect the children's language dominance.

Twins are a unique subgroup on their own. Twins may start talking later because they have little need for speech; communicating through gestures, eye-contact or simply understanding what the other twin is thinking. Parents can be concerned about early speech delay, a common occurrence in twins or multiple births. More long-term studies on twins up to the end of schooling are needed to track the language development over time and prove if the twins are affected by their late talking. Twins may have similar speech patterns, but can use language in a different ways. One can be chatty or quiet, one more precise in language use, or more attached to one language than another. We should not assume that since twins look or sound the same that they have same language patterns.

In adoptive, single, blended or step-families where children are adapting to changing family situations such as moving house, living in two homes or losing contact with family there may be some language regression as the child sorts out the emotional changes in their life. In this respect, parents should not expect too much of children in the early stages. Bilingualism is certainly an advantage, but if a child refuses or feels uncomfortable speaking one language it should be respected. Parents may need to adapt or temporarily put on hold language strategies. Children who are attending school need to have enough language to cope with the wider world of school and friends. This needs to be a priority. At home, language can be the glue that holds the family together; essential for maintaining family rituals such as eating together, sharing books, films and jokes. At the same time language choices must include the whole family and not exclude or alienate family members. It is important for these families to have a common language of communication. Step-siblings will, like any other set of siblings, chose their own preferred language, which can help facilitate friendship between the children.

As we have seen in this chapter, each family unit is a unique composition, and the advice I have given is general by nature. Each family needs to adjust depending on their needs. These special areas of bilingualism are often under-researched or non-existent in academic circles. As we have seen in the review of case studies, typical studies concentrate on two parents communicating with a young first child. Although these studies are useful and informative they do not always show the whole picture. There is a need for more real-life studies on children growing up in families where there are changing circumstances, such as parents separating or adopting a child, where serious and long-term decisions have to be made on language maintenance.

Further reading on special cases

Angelina Jolie/Brad Pitt: On WWW at http://en.wikipedia.org/wiki/Angelina_Jolie. Accessed 15.3.10.

Baker, C. (2007) *A Parents' and Teachers' Guide to Bilingualism* (3rd edn). Clevedon: Multilingual Matters.

Bowen, C. (1999) Twins development and language. On WWW at http://www.speech-language-therapy.com/mbc.htm. Accessed 15.3.10.

Brazelton, T.B. and Sparrow, J.D. (2005) *Understanding Sibling Rivalry: The Brazelton Way*. MA: De Capo Press.

Caldas, S.J. (2006) *Raising Bilingual-Biliterate Children in Monolingual Cultures*. Clevedon: Multilingual Matters.

Crystal, D. (1987) *The Cambridge Encyclopedia of Language*. Cambridge: Cambridge University Press.

Christensen, K., Petersen, I., Skytthe, A., Herskind, A-M., McGue, M. and Bingley, P. (2006) Comparison of academic performance of twins and singletons in adolescence: Follow-up study. *British Medical Journal* 333, 1095 (25 November 2006).

Dale, P., Simonoff, E., Bishop, D., Eley, T., Oliver, B., Price, T., Purcell, S., Stevenson, J. and Plomin, R. (1998) Genetic influence on language delay in two-year-old children. *Nature Neuroscience* 1, 324–8.

Garcia-Mendoza, V. (2008) What led us to these doors: Our family's journey of bilingualism and international adoption. *Multilingual Living* July/August, 26–31.

Harris, J.R. (2006) *No Two Alike Human: Nature and Human Individuality*. New York: W.W. Norton & Co.

Horney, R. (2003) Bilingualism and adoption. 'Queries' section of *The Bilingual Family Newsletter* 20 (1), 6.

Laversuch, I.M. (2004a) International adoption and bilingualism. *The Bilingual Family Newsletter* 21 (3), 6/7.

Laversuch, I.M. (2004b) Speaking the language of the enemy. *The Bilingual Family Newsletter* 21 (4), 1–4.

Livingstone, T. (2005) *Child of Our Time*. London: Bantam Books.

Majakari, N. (2006) In pursuit of my Finnish identity. *The Bilingual Family Newsletter* 23 (1), 6.

Martin, T. (2003) Multicultural adoption. 'Letters' section of *The Bilingual Family Newsletter* 20 (3), 2.

Obied, V. (2009) How do siblings shape the language environment in bilingual families? *International Journal of Bilingual Education and Bilingualism* 12 (6), 705–720.

Plomin, R. (1990) *Nature and Nurture: An Introduction to Human Behavioral Genetics.* CA: Brooks/Cole.

Schuller, M. (2002) The language acquisition of twins and twin language. Paper from seminar: 'Language Acquisition in its Developmental Context.' Accessed 24.11.08. On WWW at www.grin.com (Dokument No: V68267).

Tomosello, M., Mannle, S. and Kruger, A.C. (1986) Linguistic environment of 1- to 2-year-old twins. *Developmental Psychology* 22 (2), 169–178.

Trouton A., Spinath, F.M. and Plomin, R. (2002) Twins Early Development Study (Teds): A Multivariate, Longitudinal Genetic Investigation of Language, Cognition and Behavior Problems in Childhood. *Twin Research and Human Genetics* 5(5), 444–448.

Twinslist: http://www.twinslist.org/bilingfaq.htm (website for families with twins).

Viding, E.M., Spinath, F.M., Price, T.S., Bishop, D.V.M., Philip, S., Dale, P. and Plomin, R. (2004) Genetic and environmental influence on language impairment in 4-year-old same-sex and opposite-sex twins. *Journal of Child Psychology and Psychiatry* 45 (2), 315–325.

Wright, L. (1999) *Twins: Genes, Environment and the Mystery of Identity.* London: Wiedenfield & Nicolson.

Zuer-Pearson, B. (2008) *Raising a Bilingual Child.* New York: Living Language/Random House.

Note: For more on bilingual twins see Irene & Lisa in *Family Profiles* at the end of the book. For more on adopted bilingual siblings see Jenifer & Vicky in *Family Profiles* at the end of the book.

Chapter 9

Five Themes on Family Language Patterns

In this chapter I present the five main themes of this book – language preference, home–school transition, evolving strategies, different personalities and sibling language use. These wide topics naturally overlap to create a fascinating linguistic environment in the bilingual or multilingual home. I have found that regardless of the parents' linguistic wishes or preferences, the children choose to use one or two languages between them. This can increase or decrease use of one or two languages. Over time, language use between siblings adapts to suit the pragmatic needs of each child. As we have seen in the studies and from parent's experiences language use can have highs and lows, often linked to outside factors, such as school or friends who can strongly affect a child's perception of their bilingualism. In many homes the language evolution is subtle, and parents may not be even aware that one language is becoming passive or excluded by siblings. These common themes appear several times and encapsulate the issues of the book.

OUR 'PREFERRED' LANGUAGE

From the survey and limited research available in this area I think that children and adolescents tend to naturally choose the language of the community or school as their language of communication. This chosen language becomes their 'preferred' language, or the one the children feel most comfortable using. This choice tended to start when one or both children started school. Another option for some siblings torn between whether to speak the mother's language, father's language or the school/ community language, and perhaps risk upsetting one parent, was mixing. Mixing could vary from odd words dropped into sentences to switching languages systematically as they changed topic of conversations. In some trilingual families the siblings chose a third, or neutral, language for their preferred language.

The preferred language is not related to parental strategies or parental preferences. In fact, I found that children could choose to effectively block a parental language and *not* speak it. However, it must be noted that a preferred language was used only between siblings in private and they usually still communicated with their parents in the appropriate language. I think parents are often unaware of how this language preference could possibly undermine their carefully planned language strategies.

Can parents rebalance language use in the home? Parents who are aware of the risk of siblings relegating a minority language to the sidelines could encourage extra minority-language time, where siblings would be encouraged, or in some cases forced, to speak together in the 'other' language. This does work in some families but depends greatly on the interest and participation of the children in such language maintenance. Parents could request that older children speak a certain language with a younger siblings or even ban use of one language between them, but I consider this strategy temporary and it is considered as unnatural by children. In the long run, the decisions made by parents on the school language and the pressure of local friends should be considered as the school environment appears to have a strong influence on siblings preferred language choices.

> Siblings make clear decisions on their preferred language use together. Their choice of language(s) is *independent* of their parent's language strategy.

HOME TO SCHOOL TRANSITION

I have observed a subtle change in language use when children start formal primary schooling around age five to seven years, depending on the country. The carefully maintained home language supported by the mother, who was the main caregiver in many families, gives way to teachers and peers as role models for the children. The language of the home was sometimes replaced by the language of school for a short time, as the child adjusted to school and the new academic demands. I think the important issue is when an older sibling goes through this transition from home to school and a younger brother or sister could be influenced by the increased input of the school language at home. This outside language use comes from school homework, reading or library books brought home from the school, new friends coming to play, watching television/using computers in the school language or the older one simply preferring to use more of the school language at home. With regular contact from school or local friends the home language balance was significantly altered. A younger sibling who wanted to join in their games would soon copy this contagious linguistic behavior of using only the school/community language and dropping a parental or minority language. This could cause the siblings to shift to using only the majority language together, or a preference to mix the two languages to suit their needs.

It's not only the primary transition which affects language; becoming a teenager is a time of change too. In high school or secondary school adolescents need to identify and fit in with their peer group friends. Teenagers might totally drop or reduce the amount of minority language they used, depending on their friends opinions and values towards bilingualism or minority language use. This could potentially cause friction between younger siblings, who were two or three years younger, and frustrated and unbalanced at their older sibling's rejection of one language. In this respect the parents may need to temporarily adjust language patterns at home.

> The important *shift* from home to school, or childhood to adolescence, can induce a change of home language or the sibling preferred choice of language.

A STRATEGY TO SUIT THE CHILDREN

One theme that I saw was that a second or third child was often the catalyst for adapting language use in the home. From a relatively controllable trio of parent-parent-child the family now has to accommodate a subgroup of two or more children who can make decisions independently of parent's linguistic wishes. With a second or third child, I found some parents become stricter with the children about using the 'wrong' language. On the other hand, some parents began to tolerate more mixing by their children and decided that it was better that the children at least used some of the minority language. Seeing that one child was not speaking enough of a minority language parents might choose to try a *minority-language-at-home* strategy instead of *OPOL*, or change the school language. These are all decisions to be made within the family and I recommend families to not feel obliged to stick to one strategy if it is not working.

The parents we heard about in the book often adjusted their strategies with a second child, often by necessity as their family situation changed. Bilingual families are often mobile and move house or school frequently, perhaps switching from a country where the mother's language is spoken everywhere to one where she is one of a handful of speakers. In other families unexpected circumstances forced an adapted family strategy; a change of home, school or family members. It's important to remember the number of international families where parents divorce, and a single parent is simply not able to maintain the original family strategy. Adoption, step-families and step-parents all introduce another family language into the mix and need sensitive adjustment in language terms.

These situations are times of change and adjustment when families can find certain language strategies out of sync with their needs. The parents I talked to often struggled to keep their languages separate themselves or to keep up with increasing demands on their second language from the school or community. Others parents using a second language or following a *non-native* approach found they just could not communicate enough with their child. I think children adapt to new language circumstances, but there is a need for some revision and consideration for languages which lack support from the community.

> With the birth of a second child, or changing circumstances, parents reassess their bilingual family and may *adapt strategies* as the family evolves.

SAME LANGUAGES, DIFFERENT CHILDREN

A bilingual or multilingual child is a fascinating mix of genes, environment and parental authority. We see this, perhaps more than even in a bilingual child, in the language use, which reflects the emerging languages in the child's world and the value and effort the child exerts. Each bilingual child has its own language history, the unique blend of where each language originates and is acquired. Nevertheless; as my research has shown, even with the same two family languages and parents following the same language strategy children can turn out differently. Every sibling can have a different approach to language, some children are very chatty and talkative, other children are shy or timid and reluctant to talk to strangers. Some children mix their languages, while others might have a speech problem such as stuttering or need help with their articulation.

Children can also be affected by factors outside the home; friends, teachers, after-school activities or interests. All of these differences add up to a family with a range of language use. I consider that this mix is positive because it gives children different models of language use. I have observed that siblings can also encourage each other and give opportunities for communication that parents might not be able to do.

A family has a natural order of first-born, second-born and last-born children. Did this affect language use? I would agree that with the first child the parents often aimed high, and expected a lot of their future bilingual child. This worked in many families with first-borns typically scoring higher on correctness and a wide range of vocabulary use in both languages. Later-born children can gain from listening in to an older child's chatter and develop a potentially more creative or imaginative use of language. Like all parenting issues, from feeding, bedtimes and education we often refine our high standards of the first baby as other children join the family. Parental attitudes appeared to evolve over time as siblings play a bigger part in bringing up later-born children. I think it is important for parents not to *expect* the same level of bilingualism within their family and acknowledge the differences in ability and attitude to language learning.

> Growing up in the same family, even with the same parental or community languages, does not lead to children having the same level of bilingualism or multilingualism. *Personality differences* and *birth order* can lead children having different language histories.

INTER-SIBLING LANGUAGE USE

I have seen that language is an important part of the close relationship between siblings. In some families this natural bond can help support a parental language and encourage more use of a minority language. The siblings observed in case studies or by parents were bonding through making up stories or creating games. Being able to share jokes, expressions and role-play together was important for a close relationship. I also think siblings need someone to 'practice' on and test out language in a safe environment. Even if it appears that parents cannot hold the tide against a strong majority language from school and community the siblings can still incorporate a minority language into their private games and role-plays, giving credence to the minority language and an important place in their imagination.

Older brothers and sisters can potentially have more influence than a parent. Some older children, particularly big sisters, took on a teaching role for younger siblings. Others would try to communicate better with the younger by only using a parental language with a younger one because they saw that the little one lacked enough vocabulary to converse. However, I found that these well-meaning older brothers and sisters can sometimes reduce the actual speaking time of a younger sibling, especially if they talk *too* much for them or over-translate.

Unfortunately, there can be situations where one sibling belittles, blocks, ignores or over-corrects another child's language. In some families a parental language was employed by an older sibling to 'boss' around a younger one, or to stand in for a parent. Some siblings 'policed' each other's language use, reminding one to use a certain language or to revert to another language when they are visiting family or a country where that language is used. In other families one sibling would consciously change language and expect other siblings to follow. This tension or friction was usually temporary and linked to children moving through different phases of childhood.

Older bilingual sibling sets or bilingual parents I talked to all reported a closeness of sharing two languages and knowing how the other child dealt with the pressure of being brought up bilingual. Their established language patterns often continued into adulthood.

> Being the only speakers of a certain language, or instinctively understanding each other in both languages, can *bond* siblings. Language use between siblings can also become *negative* when used to boss or control other siblings.

CONCLUSION

I have investigated the way siblings affect the language balance within a bilingual family. Through the cooperation and generosity of the 105 international families who completed my online survey, and the 22 case studies who took the time to answer a whole range of questions, we can see more clearly how the bilingual family works. Previous studies on bilingual families are typically about a first or only child, and have implied that bilingualism is easily achievable through parental strategies such as *OPOL* or *minority-language-at-home*. Although this may work well for young children it is not always the case with older children or those with siblings.

What can we learn from the academic case studies and hearing the experiences of these international bilingual and multilingual families? We have seen throughout this book that the particular make-up of a family can affect language use in the family in several ways. Birth order, gender, age gap, family size, individual personalities or differences all work together to create a unique sibling language environment. The parent's choice of school and country where they live can strongly influence sibling's preferred language and dominant language. In parallel to the school and community, the child's friends, social life and attachment to each language or culture can affect their bilingualism too. Siblings often have a language of preference, which is not always the language that the parents prefer. A language can be maintained or dropped between siblings, regardless of the parent's wishes. Siblings form their own kind of subset within the family; they make their own rules, create opportunities for language use apart from their parents and can force parents to change language strategies. Although parents do have an important role in establishing and supporting bilingualism I think that it is the subgroup of the siblings who chose to *use* each language.

Growing up in the same family, with the same parental or community languages does not lead to children having the same bilingual or multilingual language use. Parents often find that children can be very different from each other, and one strategy which works with one child may be inappropriate for another. Each language has a different meaning for each child and siblings can feel more or less drawn to a parental language or a community language, depending on their needs. Outside influences can also affect each child differently, and we should not underestimate the power of the siblings, the school environment and their friends on bilingualism. I think there is a need for the bilingual family to evolve over time, accepting the differences and influences each child brings to the family. More research is needed into the way all children relate to their parents and the way each child relates to his or her siblings and uses language accordingly. We need more studies on families with two or more children, taking into account sibling language use, and following through to adolescence. Parents and academics working in the field of childhood bilingualism need to acknowledge this subgroup and accept that siblings give languages life and vitality, not only the parents.

Family Profiles

Families are listed alphabetically, by the parent's first name. In some families, names of children have been changed, and an alternate name has been chosen by the family.

	Parent	*Country*	*Family Languages*	*Strategy*
1	Alice	Austria	German/Spanish/English	Trilingual Lingua Franca
2	Andrea	Germany	English/German	Non-native
3	Anne	France	French/English	Time & Place
4	Christina	Germany	English/German	OPOL
5	Claudia	France	Italian/ Flemish/French/English	OPOL & 1
6	Fabiana	Malaysia	Italian/Chinese/English	Trilingual Lingua Franca
7	Gerry	Canada	English/Spanish	OPOL
8	Huw	Wales	English/Welsh	mL@H
9	Irène	France	Korean/French	mL@H
10	Jenifer	USA	Japanese/English	Non-native
11	Josie	Germany	Chinese/German/English	Trilingual Lingua Franca
12	Lilian	USA	English/Portuguese	mL@H
13	Lisa	Israel	English/Hebrew	mL@H
14	Martina	Italy	Spanish/Italian/English	OPOL/Time & Place
15	Martine	Switzerland	French/English	OPOL
16	Nadya	UK	German/English	OPOL
17	Odile	Malaysia	French/English	OPOL
18	Tammy	UK	English/Spanish	mL@H
19	Theresa	Spain	English/Spanish	Mixed
20	Toni	UK	Catalan/German/English	OPOL & 1
21	Vicky	USA	English/French	Non-native

Alice

I think that probably the more members there are in the family, and the more the kids interact with each other, the more this helps cement their bilingualism.

Alice, an editor and writer, and her husband are a trilingual English/Spanish/German family living in Austria. Multilingualism runs in the family. Alice was brought up trilingual in Korea, speaking German at home and English at school. Alice's husband is from Ecuador and he grew up speaking Spanish and acquired English later through his studies. The couple met in America during graduate school studies, and spoke English to each other from the beginning. They lived in Ecuador for a year and moved to Austria four years ago. Their daughter, Isabella, is five and their son, Dominik is two and a half years old. Isabella usually speaks English with her brother. Alice started off with the OPOL strategy. However, a change of country meant a change of language strategy at home, as Alice explains, 'When Isabella was born we lived in Ecuador and decided to use the OPOL method, with me speaking German and my husband Spanish. We kept English for communication between ourselves. This worked very well for as long as we lived in Ecuador. Then we moved to Austria, where the majority language is German. We stuck to our method for 2 years, until I realized that my daughter was overexposed to German. She got German from kindergarten and then all day from me as well. English and Spanish she would hear only after her father got home from work in the evening. Even though it was clear that she understood English and Spanish, she would reply only in German. This frustrated my husband, who, with his limited German skills at that time, felt he could not really communicate with Isabella'.

Alice and her husband decided to switch to another strategy – *Trilingual – Lingua Franca.* The plan was to reinforce English by declaring it a 'family language'; at home they would all speak English together. German was reserved for the community. Her husband spoke Spanish when interacting on a one-on-one basis with the children. Expecting problems with the new method of communicating with their children Alice and her husband found that the children reacted very well to the change. Alice reports, 'Isabella actually seemed to like the fact that we spoke English with her directly. This helped her activate English and we could include her in our conversations. Two years later, she converses in English with both of us, as well as with her little brother. She even insists that I speak English with her in the presence of her German-speaking friends when I pick her up from Kindergarten. Dominik was about one year old when I switched to English with him and things went well. His first words were in English, and it is clear that English dominates'.

On siblings and bilingualism, Alice comments, 'I used to think that I spent more time with my first-born, interacting and speaking more with her than with my youngest child, and she got a lot more language-input from me. I then realized that my daughter is playing a lot with her little brother – in English! So he is actually exposed to a lot more language variety than when my daughter was his age. Isabella had only us as language models, whereas Dominik is getting English from his parents *and* his sibling'.

Alice Lapuerta edited the *Multilingual Living Magazine*, an online magazine linked to the Multilingual Living website: www.multilingualliving.com

Andrea

> *Cherish and share the love you feel for that language/culture. Let everybody know how important the language/culture/country is to you.*

Andrea, a German linguist and translator, lived in England for nine years and speaks fluent English. Her daughter, Melanie, was born in England in 1992. Andrea moved back to Munich when Melanie was seven years old with her new German partner, Rainer, an engineer. Andrea and Rainer have two children together, Lena, age six, and Finlay, who is four. They follow a *non-native* strategy, with Andrea speaking English to her children, although the parents also speak English when the kids are present. Andrea explained, 'In the UK I spoke only German to Melanie, and when Melanie would speak to me in English I would say I didn't understand.' After moving back to Germany Andrea changed strategies to support Melanie's bilingualism. Andrea explained her reasons, saying, 'After moving to Germany, I decided to speak English to keep practicing it. Rainer always spoke German with Melanie.' However, over time Melanie's language use became more German-dominated. Andrea and Melanie usually speak German together these days, since Melanie said she preferred to use German with her mother. Nevertheless, Andrea still speaks in English to the younger children.

When Lena was born, an important decision on language use in the family was taken; the siblings would help encourage English use in the home. Melanie was asked to speak in English to Lena and help her learn to speak English. Andrea notes 'Lena used English until she was about three and a half. After six months in Kindergarten she would answer in German. Lena now speaks German to her parents but she still speaks English with her brother'. The third child, Finlay, had both his mother and two sisters as language models, although Andrea had to keep an eye on sibling language use, as Andrea says, 'If Lena would speak German to Finlay, I would point it out and say that she should speak English otherwise Finlay would not learn to speak English properly'. Now Finlay speaks English with his family and German is his weaker language, despite the fact that he has been attending a German-speaking nursery for two years.

On bringing up children with a non-native language Andrea comments, 'Do not necessarily switch languages for the benefit of speakers of the majority language. Tell people why you stick to your language and keep speaking it (you might want to say it again in the majority language, if necessary). People will understand and not think you are being impolite'. She adds, 'Don't be discouraged, it is difficult at times and hard work but your consistency will pay off in the end!'

Andrea writes a blog on non-native parenting: http://non-native-parenting. blogspot.com/

Anne

If you have difficulties in learning one language, it is even more difficult to learn two.

Anne, a former procurement manager, and her husband, Didier, a HR Director, are both French and live in Paris, France. They lived as expatriates in Bejing, China for two years and Kuala Lumpur in Malaysia for two years. They have three sons, Benjamin, 10, Antoine, 8 and Anael, 6. Benjamin and Antoine were born in France and moved to Beijing when they were, respectively, three and a half and one and half years old. Anne and Didier both speak excellent English and were keen to encourage their young children to become bilingual. At home the family mainly spoke French together and English with expatriate friends. They also had a Chinese-speaking maid/nanny working for them. Benjamin was already speaking French fluently, so following a *Time & Place* strategy Anne enrolled Benjamin in an English-language Montessori school. Benjamin enjoyed the Montessori school and did well so Anne enrolled Antoine in the same school when he was two and a half years old, but soon found that his mixed language use was causing problems. Anne reports, 'Three months later Antoine was mixing three languages all the time (out of three words in the same sentence, one was English, one Chinese, one French). When he could not pronounce one sound he would use the Chinese equivalent (e.g. the French 'je' as 'wo' because it was much easier for him). He completely ignored French grammar at that time'.

On their arrival in Kuala Lumpur, for Didier's new post, the family had to find schools for the two older boys, now aged five and three. They chose an English-language International school for Benjamin and a French-language school for Antoine. Anne explains their decision to follow two different school systems, 'When we moved to Malaysia we decided that Benjamin would stay in an English school and that Antoine needed to go to French school in order to speak at least one language correctly. The family language took priority'. Anne explained that Antoine needed speech therapy to be able to pronounce 'ch', 'j', 'gr', 'tr'. She remembered, 'Learning how to use French verbs was a nightmare for him. Speaking was difficult for him and he was simply not able to learn more than one language at the same time'. In retrospect, Anne noted that Antoine might have been overshadowed by his big brother, 'I do believe that Antoine felt, at that time, that Benjamin found it quite easy to speak two different languages. In front of his bigger brother Antoine had to fight to be able to speak'.

The family moved back to Paris in 2006 and all three children are now in local schools. Antoine and Anael both completed courses of speech therapy successfully and now speak French as per their age. Anne has organized a private tutor to speak English to Benjamin and Antoine and they have regular contact with some

English-speaking friends from Malaysia. Anne concludes 'You have children who need speech therapy and for those bilingualism is even a more difficult challenge.' She has not been put off by her experience though and plans to enroll Benjamin in a bilingual school.

Christina

> *We found that already having one bilingual child helped to reinforce our goal. Our older son acted as a 'helper' to teach his younger brother English.*

Christina, an ESL teacher and translator, lives in a small town close to Hannover in Northern Germany. She is Canadian and married to Bernhard, a German engineer. They have two sons, Tom, 15 and John, 12. The family follows the OPOL strategy; each speaking their own language to the children. Christina and her husband speak German together. Christina says that the OPOL method was successful in the their situation, 'OPOL worked exceptionally well for our situation and was really the only option available since my husband is not that proficient in English and would have felt uncomfortable speaking to the children in a non-native language. We were very strict in using OPOL both inside and outside the house, not matter who was present, and it has paid off'.

On sibling language use, Christina comments, 'The boys did start out speaking exclusively English to each other when they were small but now converse in German since starting school. They have attended public pre-school, elementary school and now secondary school here with the school language always being German'. The boys are close and although there are some differences in their language use they support each other. The older boy helped to 'reinforce' the bilingualism in the family and taught his younger brother. As Christina comments, 'Our younger son tends to mix his languages more than his older brother ever did, but it has worked out fine, and his big brother was often there to help him find the right words or remind him to only use one language at a time'. Christina concludes: 'The first child may get more intensive language input since the parents do not have to divide up their attention between two or more children, but other children have the advantage of being able to learn from their siblings'.

Christina's blog: http://justcallmemausi.blogspot.com

Claudia

> *We are a truly European family!*

Claudia, a marketing communications specialist, is Italian. Her husband, Philippe, a director in a consulting firm, is from Belgium and speaks Dutch. The couple has been living in Paris, France for the last seven years and both parents are quadrilingual. They have two sons, Milo, four and a half, and two-year-old Zeno. The family is composed of four languages, as Claudia explains, 'We are raising our children multilingual – Italian, Dutch, French (active) and English (passive). We have been using strictly OPOL when we speak to the children, and my husband and I speak English to each other at home'. The French language comes from the community where they live, so the family language pattern is *OPOL & 1*. Milo and Zeno have been looked after by French speaking nannies since they were babies. Milo has attended a local *crèche* since he was 2½ years old, where French was the predominant language. He is now in *école maternelle* (preschool)'.

Claudia is happy with the OPOL strategy, as she says, 'We keep sticking to OPOL and it gives good results. It certainly makes things easier and it reassures the kids. When I tried, just for fun, to say a few sentences in Dutch (my husband's language), Milo was shocked and asked me not to do that anymore. He also did not like me speaking French when he was younger; he tolerates it when we are in the presence of French people, but at home he wants me to read books in Italian, sing in Italian. He is interested in learning English, so from time to time he asks me how do we say this and that in English, or read some English books we have'.

On siblings and bilingualism, Claudia comments on the perspective of her younger son, Zeno, who has a different language model to his big brother, Milo. Claudia explains, 'The second-born child has one more individual to look up to; the older sibling who speaks *all of the languages involved at once*. This definitely has an impact. There are three adults who speak each a different language (mum, dad, nanny/teacher), and there's a little brother who uses all three. It must be puzzling somehow'. Claudia thinks this could make a difference to Zeno's language learning pattern and she is recording their day to day speech in her blog.

'Of Languages Mixing: When OPOL is harder with the second child', *Multilingual Living* (Winter 2009: 26/27)

Claudia's blog: http://multitonguekids.blogspot.com

Fabiana

We are a mixed-culture and mixed-language family.

Fabiana is Italian and her husband, Michael, a lawyer, is a Malaysian with Chinese heritage. Both parents are fluent in English and have been living in Kuala Lumpur, Malaysia since 1993. They have three daughters, Martina, 10, Natalia, 9, Arianna, 6 and one son, one-year-old Thomas. Fabiana describes her family as a unique blend of Italian, Chinese, English and Bahasa Malaysia. Their language strategy at home is *Trilingual – Lingua Franca*. Fabiana explains, 'Between the two of us we speak English. However, Michael and I made an effort in learning each other's language, in fact, Michael speaks fluent Italian and I am learning Mandarin'. Fabiana speaks Italian to her children and Michael speaks English to the girls. However, with the birth of their fourth child Michael has started speaking more Mandarin, especially to the baby. This does not pose a problem in this multilingual family as Fabiana notes, 'We all understand my husband when he talks to the baby (in Chinese) and the girls like to sing Chinese songs to their brother'. Fabiana explains why her husband changed his language strategy as home, 'We chose the OPOL strategy because we wanted to be able to be completely comfortable in expressing ourselves with the children. Excited with our success in making our girls bilingual, we decided to introduce Mandarin with Thomas, so that the Chinese element will also find more relevance in our family. I ask the girls to use Italian to their little brother, rather than English, and they sometimes enthusiastically, sometimes reluctantly, try to do so. They understand and feel the importance of it'.

Their daughters naturally switch languages and behaviour according to the person they are talking to. The girls are also learning a fourth language at school. Fabiana explains 'The girls go to an international school where they speak English and study Bahasa Malaysia as second language. They also have been taking Mandarin classes for years and they are just learning to converse in this language. Among themselves they use English'. Fabiana observes, 'All three girls are fluent in both languages, but it seems that Martina has a wider vocabulary than the sisters. In fact, her Italian is much better than many Italian kids of her age, even though we visit Italy only once a year. Natalia and Arianna's Italian is less grammatically correct than Martina's. We noticed that as soon as they step outside home their social language becomes English. They stopped using Italian among themselves as they used to and it became harder for Arianna to speak it. We have been sticking to OPOL, and Arianna slowly managed to develop very good Italian, along with her English. They are now slowly learning to write and read Italian and in this case the birth order is reversed. Arianna has a better grasp of the Italian phonetic and spelling, Natalia follows immediately after and Martina instead tends to apply English phonetics to her Italian reading and writing'.

Gerry

Parents should primarily be sensitive to the needs of the individual child and later consider the greater good of the family as well.

Gerry is a Canadian Medical/Scientific translator and freelance writer and her husband was born in Mexico. The family lives in Kingston, Ontario. Both parents are bilingual and individually speak their native languages with the children. They usually speak English with each other, unless in a Spanish speaking environment, or in the company of guests who do not understand English, in which case, they use Spanish. The couple has four children – three boys born in 1994, 1996, 2000, and a daughter born in 2002. The siblings use Spanish at home with their father. Gerry says 'We have naturally and primarily, by default, used the OPOL strategy with all of our children'. Like many bilingual families they have changed countries and school systems frequently. The family returned to Canada in 2007, after living in Mexico and British Columbia. Gerry notes that their schools have also changed numerous times, due to the family moving house and academic necessity.

Initially, their two eldest children attended an English immersion primary school in Mexico. In Canada, they took advantage of a local French language immersion school near to their home for their two school-aged children. The children then transferred to a regular English curriculum after another move to an area where French immersion was not available. The family returned to Mexico where the three school-aged boys attended a Spanish immersion school with English as a second language. A brief hiatus from the school system allowed Gerry to home-school the youngest children using a bilingual approach. Later, they transferred the four children to a two-way immersion (English and Spanish) school and then, to a pre-dominately Spanish-language school where English was taught as a second language. Currently, all the children are attending an English-language school with core French daily.

The family is sensitive to each child's particular needs and have changed strategies when needed, as Gerry explains: 'Our third son was slightly speech delayed and so my husband began to use one language (English) with him alone, in order to facilitate his grasp on the language'. At the time English was used at home and in society. Gerry adds, 'The two older boys were in French immersion school and my husband had been speaking Spanish with all of the boys at home. So, when we perceived that the single language use was successful for our youngest child we went back to the OPOL method, which helped us integrate more Spanish into his daily life. After moving to Mexico, where our language of major communication immediately switched to Spanish, we observed his very quick integration into the language and culture; thanks to the exposure we feel he had received by using the OPOL method in Canada'.

On siblings and bilingualism, Gerry says: 'If the first-born child is raised in a bilingual environment, the chances are higher for subsequent children to be exposed to, offered or provided with, the same or further bilingual opportunities. Younger siblings may have a much richer exposure to dual language use and thus, have an easier time being or becoming bilingual among the group. In our particular case, the stimulus has been akin to positive feedback, and with each child welcomed into the family, the enjoyment and use of languages has increased tremendously; so much that we have a group interest in many other languages and can also appreciate other cultures to a much greater extent as a family'.

'Bi-cultural parenting: Two Culture Homes', *Multilingual Living* (Nov/Dec 2006: 42/43)

'Using two or more languages at home: One family's journey', *Multilingual Living* (March/April 2007: 88/89)

Gerry also contributes to the Canadian Culture website: www.canadianculture.com

Huw

Language acquisition and retention are extremely complex processes influenced by a rich variety of factors.

Huw, a University lecturer, and his wife, both in their early sixties, live in Gwynedd, Wales. They are Welsh speakers, but were not brought up in a strong Welsh environment. As Huw says, 'In my case the language at home when I was a child was normally English, principally because we lived in an anglicized area of Wales and Welsh then did not have the social cachet attached to it that it enjoys today'. Before starting a family the couple spoke English together. After the birth of their first child, a daughter, they made 'the conscious decision to change the language of the home to Welsh'. When their son was born two years later they kept going with their family language strategy of *minority-language-at-home*, to maintain the Welsh language. This was a success and Huw reports proudly that 'Both our children are now in their early thirties and have a high level of bilingual skills. They both did well across the school curriculum. Our daughter is now a doctor, our son a radio producer'. The children accepted their parents' Welsh language use and found it curious that their parents at one time spoke English to each other. As their father notes, 'There are occasions, in the presence of non-Welsh speakers, when we have to converse with our children in English. I sometimes find that difficult, as the conversation can appear to be somewhat artificial if not stilted. But I'm getting used to it!'

Huw recounts his own linguistic history, which influenced his decision to speak only Welsh to his children, saying 'I was one of two children, my sister being four years younger than me. We both attended Welsh-medium infant schools but were switched at the age of seven to English-medium education. Welsh-medium education was still in its early days at that time. We both spoke English at home and with each other and most of our friends. My sister identified strongly with the English pop scene, qualified as a nurse and followed her career in England. Her skills in Welsh are correspondingly low. I followed an academic path and at university in England consciously identified myself with the strong language movement then gaining momentum in Wales and with the cultural/political links associated with the language (e.g. Welsh literature; pacifism). Consequently, I became involved with a number of Welsh-speaking circles of colleagues that helped me to affirm my Welsh identity, including my language skills'. Huw concludes 'My gut feeling is that the first sibling has a natural "advantage" but that this is necessarily qualified by a whole range of other influences, which have to be taken together'.

Irene

Each family must find what works best for them.

Irene, a photographer and freelance writer, and her husband, Yoon-Seok, live in Paris, France. Her parents immigrated to France soon after they got married in 1975 and

Irene was born in France. She grew up bilingually, speaking both French and Korean. Her husband came to France 17 years ago and speaks both French and Korean. Their twin sons, Sean and Will, were born in 2002. The family follows the *minority-language-at-home* strategy as Irene says: 'We both speak Korean to our children and they respond in French. Sean and Will speak French together and at school'. Like many children in bilingual families, the issue is how to keep the minority language (Korean) active and in use. Irene says that Sean and Will are now old enough to understand that their parents are both fluently bilingual and can speak either language, but French tends to be their default language. The twins often reply to their parents' Korean in French, a scenario often seen in bilingual families.

Irene describes the family's language use, 'Our twin boys talk French at school and with each other. When we talk to them in Korean they respond in French. I think it's because they know we understand French. When they are around family members who do not speak French though, they will try to talk Korean. We think they understand about 90% of what we tell them in Korean'. Having being brought up with two languages in a *minority-language-at-home* environment Irene has experience of bilingualism first-hand. However, she was an only child and now finds it harder to influence the language choices her five-year-old twin boys make. Irene comments: 'The *minority-language-at-home* strategy worked well for me when I was little because I was an only child. It's harder to apply it with my twins because they talk to each other in French and will obviously not make the effort to talk in Korean'.

Irene's blog: http://irenenam.squarespace.com/

Jenifer

There is a sense of shared history and a shared secret language between our children. I would think in the future it would create a strong bond between them.

Jenifer teaches Linguistics and her husband, Andrew, teaches Japanese History at the University of North Texas. They are both American and live in Texas, Jenifer and Andrew both speak fluent Japanese and have lived in Japan. They are bringing up their three adopted children, Lachlan, 9, Kiki, 5 and baby Case Kaye, bilingually with English and Japanese. The family follows a *non-native* approach, with both parents speaking Japanese to their children. In America the children speak English together. Jenifer recounts how it all started, 'Our first son, Lachlan, was adopted at birth, and came to Japan with us when he was three months old. He started going to Japanese daycare at age nine months, and stayed there until we returned to the US when he was about 18 months old. When he was about two years old I made the decision to speak only Japanese with him. My husband also spoke Japanese mostly to him. We returned to Japan when Lachlan was two and a half. He began going to a Japanese-language full-time daycare/preschool immediately'.

Jenifer recalls that the adoption of their second child, Kiki, when Lachlan was four, strengthened the family's decision to bring up their children bilingually. She says,

'Our second child, Kiki, was born in Japan. Kiki was just one when she was adopted, and had lived in a Japanese orphanage until then. When we adopted her I told the child welfare office I would speak Japanese to her. It became less of just a game and more a feeling that I could help her retain her ethnic identity so that if she ever wanted to return to Japan to live she could'.

Although the family left Japan soon after and returned to Texas they were able to keep up their Japanese contact. With regular vacations of two to three months in Japan each summer the children were able to attend local schools. On the question of their choice to bring up their children bilingually Jenifer says, 'I would say people think it's cool. There have been maybe one or two comments about speaking a "secret language" by my father-in-law, and generally we find it much harder to keep speaking to the kids if we are staying with family, but I think people are supportive. Lachlan was a late talker and my sister suggested it was the bilingualism, but I'd done enough reading of the literature at that point to know it wasn't true'.

Josie

I think birth order affects bilingualism … to the extent that the eldest sibling proba-bly determines which language is dominant.

Josie, a former lawyer, is a trilingual Malaysian. Her husband, Thomas, a lawyer, is German and speaks English. Josie and Thomas have three boys, Niklas, 12, Tobias, 8, and four-year-old Lukas. Josie says 'My husband and I met at university in England and English was initially our common language'. The family has lived in Germany, Kuala Lumpur and Singapore and for the last two and half years they have lived in Bensberg, near Cologne in Germany. Josie has a multilingual language history, as she explains, 'My mother tongue is Chinese – a dialect called Hokkien. I also speak some Cantonese, the dialect one needs to get by in the Chinese community in Kuala Lumpur, but my Mandarin is very poor. I learnt Malay and English as a second language at school. English is the language in which I communicate best. I also speak German and I would say that this is now my second best language'.

The parents initially followed the OPOL strategy with Niklas, with some third language input from the community and grandparents. Josie recalls, 'In the begin-ning we lived in Malaysia and I spoke English to Niklas and my husband spoke German. We never mixed the languages when we spoke to Niklas, although between us we used both languages interchangeably. My parents spoke Mandarin to him from birth in the hope that Niklas would grow up trilingual. When he was three months old we moved to Germany and due to the infrequency in which my parents saw him it was hard to keep Chinese going. Although he first learnt to count in Mandarin and could say a few words today Niklas can no longer speak any Mandarin'.

The family moved to Singapore in 1999. All three boys went to the German Kindergarten and School, where the language of instruction was German. However,

English was also spoken in kindergarten as usually one teacher in each kindergarten group was Singaporean and spoke English. Josie remarks 'When we lived in Singapore, we encouraged the children to speak German to each other'. When the family returned to Germany five years later Josie found it hard to keep English active in the home, as she says, 'We tried to reverse it after returning to Germany, but the children could not be persuaded to speak English between themselves. Only Lukas, who is four, will sometimes still say something to his brothers in English, but that is increasingly rare'. The family now follows a more *Trilingual – Lingua Franca* approach, as Josie concludes, 'German has become the main language spoken in our family. I continue to speak to the boys only in English and Lukas is the only one who still communicates with me in English. Thomas and I speak English to each other occasionally'. However, the children have not forgotten English, as Josie notes, 'Niklas has no problem communicating in English when he has to. Tobias struggles with English and conversations on the phone with my parents and sisters are monosyllabic on his part. But after two weeks or so in Malaysia during the summer holidays, it does get easier for him'.

Lilian

I think being flexible is very important. It is equally important not to lose focus.

Lillian and Kleberg are Brazilian and have been living in America for 11 years. They speak Portuguese at home are both fluent in English. Their two sons, Kelvin, five, and Linton, three, were born in America. The family follows a *minority-language-at-home* strategy (Portuguese). Lilian says that they try to encourage as much use of Portuguese at home as they can, but there are times when the majority language is used too, as she explains, 'Our strategy was speaking Portuguese at home. However, when our oldest boy became fluent in English he began to speak English to us, and without thinking about it we replied. Or once in a while we have to speak English while helping him with homework. It's also possible that we read to him in English, although he did not like that before and the youngest still does not – we translate any books that are in English for them.'

Kelvin started kindergarten last fall while Linton stays at home with Lilian and their Brazilian grandparents who care for them at home. The family also attends a Brazilian church regularly. On language, Lilian says, 'Kelvin was mostly monolingual, in Portuguese, until he was four and began to learn English from playing online games (PBS kids) and watching TV shows (Sesame Street and other public television shows) as well as DVDs'. Regarding her strategy, Lilian comments, 'It would be easier to enforce the *minority-language-in-the-home* "rule" with only one child since children value more what their peers (siblings or other children) do and what language they speak than their parents. My youngest is much more interested in speaking English than Portuguese because of his brother and his friends'. Lilian is concerned about how to keep Portuguese active in the home, when her boys spend more time in outside activities. She says, 'I'm aware that if I'm not careful and start to speak English more frequently with my sons, Portuguese may fall by the wayside. I still worry about the fact that once my youngest becomes fluent in English they are very likely going to speak in English between them and what's going to become of their fluency in Portuguese?'

'Afraid of English', *Multilingual Living* (Sept/Oct 2006: 18)

http://mamaintranslation.blogspot.com/

Lisa

I think the fact that my girls speak English between themselves helps keep it strong.

Lisa is American and her husband is Israeli and they have twin girls, Rachel and Sarah, who were born in 1994 in Israel. The family lives in Israel. In the beginning the family followed an OPOL strategy; Lisa spoke English and her husband Hebrew. The family moved to England when the girls were ten months and lived there for two years. Lisa reports, 'By the time they were about 22 months, they were using the right language for the right parent. When they started speaking in full sentences, they stopped speaking Hebrew (the minority language at the time).'

The family moved to America when the twins were three, and spent 18 months there. When they returned to Israel after their posting, Lisa observed her four-year-old daughter's reactions to now being in a country where Hebrew was the majority language, 'After taking about a month to get over the initial shock of finding out that someone other than their father spoke Hebrew, they quickly got used to speaking it'. The family also spent a year in the US when the girls were in primary school. Lisa comments 'During that time, they were in the 4th grade and attended an ESL class once a week – mainly to work on their reading and writing. Their spoken English was close to grade level.' The family now follow a *minority-language at home* strategy, which suits them all.

On the twins language use Lisa says, 'They both hate speaking/hearing mixed speech, or as we call it, "Heblish". In general, they speak English between themselves. When they were younger, if they were continuing a game they started at school, they'd switch to Hebrew'. Now Rachel and Sarah are 14 and in the 8th grade at school. According to Lisa they both read at, or above, grade level in English (the minority language). Lisa adds, 'Sarah currently attends a bilingual Hebrew-Arabic school. Even though she started in 7th grade, this awareness of the structure of language enabled her to join the regular Arabic as a Second Language class by the beginning of 8th'. Lisa concludes, 'At this point, their language skills are pretty similar. Rachel, who is more outgoing, is more likely to slip into slang, "Ya know, like," etc. in both languages. Sarah tends to be more precise; she's very aware of grammatical rules and correct usage'.

Lisa maintains the online *twinslist* community (run by the University of Southern California), which offers guidance and information to families with multiple births: http://www.twinslist.org (see Bilingual Families).

Martina

I think that the closer the children are the easier it is for them to talk.

Martina, an English teacher, is Venezuelan and married to an Italian, Nicola, a lift engineer, who speaks fluent English and Spanish. They have two daughters, Alessia, 8 and Gaia, 6. Martina is trilingual in Spanish, English and Italian and was educated in an English-language American school. The family has lived in Grado, a small town between Venice and Trieste in Italy since 1996. Their family has a trilingual strategy – a mix of OPOL for the two parental languages and *Time & Place* for English. Martina explains how each language is used in their family. 'At home I speak Spanish to my husband and he speaks Italian to me. He speaks Italian to our daughters and I speak Spanish to them'.

Alongside supporting Spanish, Martina was keen to pass on her love of English language to her daughters and began by introducing them to English-language children's programs when they were young, as she explains, 'We decided that my husband would speak in Italian and I would speak in Spanish. At the same time I bought all the Barney videotapes and songs in English I could find and I had my daughter watch only tapes in English. When Gaia was born, we continued with the Italian–Spanish (from the parents) and English thanks to TV and music. Now that they are older and understand that different people speak different languages I am trying to speak in English outside of the home too, or sometimes at home we play "pretend" games in English'.

The girls attend a local Italian school and usually speak Italian together. Martina notes that the girls are close and spend a lot of time with each other, 'Alessia and Gaia are always talking between them they speak Italian. Only after a two-month vacation in Caracas with my family, did they start to speak Spanish between them, but that changed back to Italian when we got back to Italy'. Martina is using technology and her daughter's love of singing to encourage the girl's trilingualism. She says, 'I allow them to watch cable TV and play online English phonics game, or visit websites like *Sesame Street, Clifford* or whatever they are into at the moment. We have been through the *Wiggles, Dora the Explorer* and HI 5. Now we are into *Hannah Montana, High School Musical* and *Camp Rock!*' Martina also finds songs her daughters like via YouTube, both in Spanish and English, and compiles CDs with the songs they like the most in both languages.

Martine

You should never change your strategy – stability, perseverance and continuity give a good foundation.

Martine is a French teacher. She is French and married to an Englishman, James, who is a bank manager. The family has lived in Zurich, in the German-speaking part of Switzerland, since 2007. Previously, the family lived for 14 years as expatriates in

Hong Kong and Singapore, and their two children were born there. Their daughter, Tiéphaine, is 10 and son, Xavier, is 8. Martine describes the family language pattern as OPOL, commenting: 'Our kids speak English with their father and French with me. I speak English to my husband who replies in English. He does not speak French'. In Hong Kong and Singapore, the children attended private French-language schools. However, as Martine notes 'English was the second language at the French school and was widely spoken in the community'.

The family wanted to keep English strong at home, as Martine explains, 'When we arrived in Switzerland we tried to establish that weekends should be "English speaking" but it did not work and the kids were very frustrated so we stopped and went back to our normal bilingual way of life'. In Switzerland, the children are enrolled in a French-speaking school. Martine taught French in Asia, and understands the problems some bilingual children can face in education. She says, 'I saw a few kids in Singapore who were diagnosed as "dyslexic" which was in fact not the case. Some bilingual children have difficulties learning two languages at the same time, especially with sounds and phonetics and are often misled'.

Nadya

> *Together with a group of parents in Bristol, we have set up a German Saturday School so that our children can mix with others growing up in the same way.*

Nadya, a science journalist, lives in Bristol, England with her English husband, Matthew, an electronics engineer. They have two daughters, Elicia, 5 and Charlotte, 3, who they are bringing up bilingually. Nadya's childhood was multilingual; her mother is German and her father English. As a child she lived in Germany, where her English father spoke German. The family then moved to Wales, where she attended a bilingual school and consequently learnt Welsh. Nadya remembers how she and her younger brother used German as their 'secret language' to talk together.

Nadya says, 'I am second generation bilingual, so I know first-hand the benefits of bilingualism. I am half German and married to an Englishman. So even though my two daughters are only a quarter German, I speak only German to them, even in public surrounded by English people'. Nadya feels very strongly about continuing the use of German in her family. The family follows an OPOL approach, with Nadya speaking German to her girls, and her husband English. Nadya describes herself as 'strict' about speaking German and prefers to translate English-language books into German when she reads to her daughters. She encourages the girls to hear as much German as they can through German-language television or DVDs, and visits her family in Germany.

Understanding the benefits of bilingualism she is helping other German-speaking families living in her area support the minority language too. In January 2008, together with a group of parents, Nadya helped set up a German Saturday School in Bristol, for children aged three to 12. The idea came from her experience with other young parents in German-language playgroups who found that once their children started going to primary school their German became passive and under-used, especially in terms of playing and socializing with other children. In an article written for *The Bilingual Family Newsletter* Nadya wrote that the school encouraged children to feel they can express themselves bilingually and practice using the minority language in a relaxed setting. Nadya says 'The school gives bilingual children a chance to feel normal and to feel comfortable about speaking other languages. It gives families a sense of community and a chance to get to know each other. And above all, it's a fun place to be!'

'How to set-up a Saturday School' by Nadya Anscombe.
The Bilingual Family Newsletter (2008) 25 (3)
www.schule-bristol.org
www.germansaturdayschools.co.uk

Odile

I would never dream of dropping French as I think it's a great advantage to have access to two cultures.

Odile is French and lives with her English husband, Steve, a Marketing Director for an international market research company, in Kuala Lumpur, Malaysia. They have three children, Amy, seven, Luca, five and Elliot, 20 months old. The two older children attend English language schools. The family use the OPOL strategy as Odile explains, 'Since having children we stuck to Dad speaking English and Mum French and it seems to work. My husband and I speak French at home, but while eating, for instance, the children always address him in English'. The two older children attend English-language International schools. The family also has exposure to several languages used in Malaysia (Bahasa Malaysia, Chinese and Tamil) through their links to the local community. Odile has volunteered her time working with an orphanage in Kuala Lumpur for over five years. She has established a friendship with a Malaysian girl with Indian heritage who is the same age as Amy, and who comes to visit the family regularly. The family also has a Tamil-speaking maid who often looks after the children.

Odile says that she is serious about language use, commenting, 'If the children get lazy with me and start introducing shorter English words or bad English translation into our conversation, I'm very strict in the sense that I make them repeat the correct word or sentence in French, sometimes several times to make sure they remember and I ask them to repeat the right thing, systematically!' However, there are some exceptions to the rule as Odile reports: 'The one thing I make allowance for sometimes is when Amy and I do maths homework, and I will say some numbers in English after I realize she's confused with the French'. Odile concludes that bilingualism is a good thing for her family, saying 'I think having the French and English cultures is what is bonding my kids and make them such good partners in everything. They stick together and I'm sure it has something to do with the fact that they speak a language no one else around them does'.

Tammy

We now sprinkle more English into the home whereas when we just had one child we were more exclusive to Spanish.

Tammy, a former financial analyst, and her husband, Frank, a crude oil trader, have lived in Surrey, England for four years. Tammy and Frank are both American and of Hispanic heritage. Tammy's family immigrated from Cuba and Frank has Mexican heritage. They have four daughters, Isabel, 8, Elena, 6, Monica, 3 and baby Nora. Tammy and her husband both speak fluent Spanish and the family follows a *minority-language-at-home* strategy, with some extra support from school for two of their children. Tammy comments, 'I think our situation is quite common, especially in the USA, where there are many immigrant groups speaking their native language and from one generation to the next the language can be lost completely. My husband and I are both first generation Americans and learned Spanish first from our families, later being educated 100% in English. We decided to speak Spanish exclusively to our children when we had our oldest daughter, Isabel, in 1999'. Tammy notes that there are several challenges to keeping Spanish active in the home. She usually talks in English with her husband, saying 'We are more comfortable speaking English to each other, as our Spanish level is conversational and at an elementary level'. Tammy and her husband also found that when Isabel was seven years old she 'surpassed their Spanish level threshold' and it became difficult for them to discuss certain abstract concepts with her in Spanish, such as religion.

The two older girls attend an American-curriculum International School. The school offers Spanish language classes to primary age children after school. Tammy clarifies, 'The purpose of these classes is for children from Spanish speaking countries to retain their language at a level where they could return to their home country and assimilate into the school system at their appropriate age level. My children do not fall under this category since we are American, and would not be living in a Spanish speaking country. But because we consider Spanish our children's first language, they allow us to participate in the program'. However, Tammy has noticed that 'Isabel has become so comfortable with her main school language, English, that she does not want to challenge herself and continue speaking Spanish at home with her parents whom she knows understand English'. Tammy has found that the younger girls heard their older sisters speaking English to each other and preferred that language. She adds, 'Baby Nora is almost one and I am afraid will not speak Spanish at all despite our trying!' Nevertheless, Tammy is doing all she can to support their family's language and cultural heritage for her four daughters.

Theresa

I think the parents need to play an active role in getting the kids to use the minority language; otherwise it's just too easy to go over to the dominant language.

Theresa, an EFL teacher, is an American born to Dutch parents. She has been living in Pamplona, Spain for over 15 years. Theresa is bilingual (English/Spanish) and can read and understand Dutch too. Her Spanish husband, Jesús, is a professor at the Universidad Publica de Navarra, and speaks fluent English. The couple have three daughters, Carmen, 13, Rocío, 11 and Violeta, 9. The family language pattern is *mixed*, as Theresa says 'My husband and I mix English and Spanish when speaking to each other, but Spanish is dominant. I try to use mostly English with the kids, although sometimes we lapse over to Spanish. My husband speaks both to them, about equally. The kids usually reply in Spanish, although sometimes they'll switch to English.' Theresa adds 'Whenever we can, we watch movies and television shows in English, which is now much easier with digital television'.

The three girls usually use Spanish with each other, but know when to change languages as Theresa reports, 'When my mother, who doesn't speak Spanish, visits, the kids switch over to English without too much trouble'. Theresa noticed that her children have formed a strong emotional bond with her mother through the use of English, and adds 'When they are with her they tend to use English with each other as well'. Theresa notes that Carmen speaks both Spanish and English fluently and reads well in both languages. She is now learning French at school. Rocío speaks both Spanish and English but her English is less fluent. Rocío can communicate well in English, but she makes many grammatical errors. Violeta speaks mostly Spanish but can communicate at a basic level in English. Her comprehension of English is much better than her speaking skills.

The language used at the girls' bilingual school is mostly Spanish, although they have subjects taught only in English. Theresa remarks on the challenge of keeping the minority language active in the family. She says 'With two or more children, I think there is a tendency for them to use the language of the country they live in when talking to each other. Language growth in general may be stimulated by having siblings, since there are more opportunities for communication, but for second language acquisition it may be a hindrance'.

Theresa's blog: http://rainypamplona.blogspot.com/

Toni

The kids have very little contact with Catalan so I am pleasantly surprised that they actually speak the language at all.

Toni, a Water Resources Manager, lives in Birmingham, England. His wife, Natalie, a language teacher, is German and fluent in English. Natalie also speaks and understands reasonably well Italian, Catalan, French and Spanish. The couple has lived in England since the early 1990s, and they have two small children, a four-year-old daughter, Laia, and two-year-old son, Elies. They follow an OPOL + 1 strategy at home – Catalan from Toni, German from Natalie and English from the community. Toni and Natalie speak English with one another. Toni was brought up bilingually, as he recounts, 'I am a Catalan who grew up with Catalan (the community language in Catalonia) and Spanish (my parents' language). My parents spoke to me and my sister in Catalan to help us feel part of the community. I also learned English from the age of six by spending summer holidays in the UK with family friends.'

Laia attends a local English nursery school and Elies goes to an English child-minder on a part-time basis. Like many fathers in bilingual families Toni spends less time with his children than he would prefer and comments, 'In a normal week I only see my kids at the weekend, and two to three evenings for about a couple of hours each time'. Toni also notes that he is often the only 'model' of the languages, saying 'As we don't often have Catalan friends around and we only visit Catalonia for a week in the summer, they rarely hear Catalan as language spoken by anybody else but me'. At home the Catalan language is supported by DVDs, CDs and satellite television.

To counteract the low input of Catalan at home Toni set up a network of bilingual Catalan-speaking families in the United Kingdom, that meet two or three times a year for a weekend to encourage their kids to speak Catalan. On the mother's side, Natalie has set up a weekly German language playgroup in the Birmingham area. The children often spend time in Germany with Natalie's parents in a German mono-lingual environment. The children also have a collection of German DVDs and CDs at home. The family is planning to move to Catalonia soon where both children will be starting school in Catalan. Toni adds, 'Once their Catalan is up to speed we will decide whether to send them to a German school. As for English, even though we will continue to use it as a couple, we will also have to think how to best support this language'.

Catalan-speakers in UK website: http://groups.google.com/group/families-catalanes-uk

Vicky

Our children are close enough in age that they share much of the kaleidoscope and ever changing frame of reference of language development.

Vicky, a former diplomat and volunteer with children's charities, and her husband, Nick, a diplomat, have lived in London, England for four years. They are both origi-nally from America, and have lived as expatriates in Madagascar, Ethiopia and Kuwait. They have two children, Annis, 10 and William, 9. Both children were adopted; their daughter from America at birth and their son at age seven weeks from Madagascar. Vicky describes their family as an international one, noting that their children have already lived in four countries.

In terms of language strategies, the family follows a *non-native* approach, with the father speaking French to his children. Nick spent the first seven years of his school life in France and felt it was important to raise his children bilingually with the French language. His early experiences were very strong as Vicky says, 'He still automatically counts in French!' Vicky was keen to pass on this French connection to their children, although Nick was initially dubious about speaking his second language to his children, but he now sees bilingualism as a 'given'. Vicky recounts, 'My husband has always and consistently spoken French with both children, and English with me'. Vicky always speaks English with her husband and with the children, although she understands all the French spoken. However, the family is flexible and will adapt their language use, for example, if the children are playing with non-French-speaking friends.

Both children were enrolled in French-language *Lycèe Français* preschools in the countries they lived in, but now attend local English language schools in London. Together Annis and William speak English, usually with an American accent, although Vicky notes that their English is more 'British' these days. On the question of adoption and bilingualism, Vicky thinks that her family and friends have been very supportive. She comments, 'Some eyebrows were raised initially, but nothing really critical. The only time I thought it may have been a mistake was for the couple of months when William stuttered (around age two), but that quickly passed'. Vicky says that other families in the same position should think of it as a gift to their children and help them discover the joy of languages.

Appendix 1
Summary of Strategies

There are six groups of language strategies that are commonly used to describe bilingual families. These categories come from academic work done in the field of bilingualism, and I have added some categories in line with the family strategies I found while researching this book. Each strategy has its positive side, and in some cases there can be a negative effect too. Some strategies are stricter and depend on the parents choosing which language is used at a certain time, while other strategies allow for family members to make their own decisions about which language they use. Readers should bear in mind that the categorization of parental language/child language/location and school language are general and do not necessarily apply to all families. The following chart shows a summary of the basic characteristics of each strategy (highlighted in gray).

ONE-PARENT–ONE-LANGUAGE (OPOL)

Each parent speaks their own language to the children

If you and your partner each speak *only* your first language to your children you are probably following the OPOL approach. This is one of the most well-known strategies and was used by several parent-linguists mentioned in Chapter 1 (see Werner Leopold and Traute Taeschner). In general, OPOL tends to be more popular among European families and is often quoted in articles and books on bilingualism as the 'best' way to give a child a chance of being fully bilingual. This has never been proved however, and remains more of a myth than reality, although OPOL is well suited to young children and is a good way for parents to keep using their own languages while living in a country where their language is not supported. Almost 40% of the families in my study preferred the OPOL strategy. There are some varieties of OPOL, depending on the language choices the parents make and the language of the community where they live.

OPOL (majority)

One parent speaks language A to children
One parent speaks language B to children

Together the parents speak Language A
The family lives in country using Language A

Children most likely attend school in Language A
Siblings will most likely use Language A together

Positive: Establishes early language distinctions. Allows B-speaking parent to keep on using his or her language (even if other parent does not understand it).

Negative: Language-B speaker lacks support and their language can become passive over time.

OPOL (minority)

One parent speaks Language A to children
One parent speaks Language B to children

Together the parents speak Language B
The family lives in country using Language A

Children most likely go to school using Language A
Siblings most likely to use mostly Language A (and some B)

Positive: Establishes early language distinctions and allows B-speaking parent to keep on using his or her language with another adult.

Negative: The Language B-speaking parent can lack support from community and feel pressurized to use more Language A in public.

OPOL (mixed)

One parent speaks Language A to children
One parent speaks Language B to children

Together the parents speak Language A & B
The family lives in country using Language A

Children most likely go to school using Language A
Siblings most likely to use mostly Language A (and some B)

Positive: Like other OPOL choices, establishes early language distinctions and allows B-speaking parent to keep on using his or her language with another adult.

Negative: As in the OPOL minority language strategy, the Language B-speaking parent can lack support from community and feel pressurized not to mix or use his or her language in public.

OPOL + 1: Two parental languages and one language from the country where they currently live

One parent speaks Language A to children
One parent speaks Language B to children

Together the parents speak Language A or B

The family lives in country using Language C

Children most likely attend school in Language C
Siblings will most likely use Language C (& some A or B)

Positive: The children generally become trilingual.

Negative: Hard to support one or both parental languages without extra support.

For more details on OPOL parenting strategies see my book: *Language Strategies for Bilingual Families: The One Parent One Language Approach* (2004).

MIXED LANGUAGE USE: BILINGUAL AND MULTILINGUAL

A mélange of parental languages or parent/country languages

In many bilingual families *mixing* is a natural and normal way of communicating. Families who mix often don't see it as a strategy – it is just how things are. In fact, 40% of the respondents in my survey said they regularly mixed languages, either with their children or their partner. Families who mix often live in parts of the world where mixing is a common practice. This might be an officially bilingual country such as Switzerland, Singapore, Wales or Luxembourg. The family might live near a border area of two countries, where traditionally trade between the two countries has made bilingualism the norm. Mixing is common in Asia, India, Middle East and neighboring countries in Europe. For mixing to work effectively *both* parents need to be bilingual, or at least have a good understanding of each other's languages. Mixing was often dismissed as academics as giving children a bad example. Consequently, it has been rather under-researched, compared to the body of work on OPOL. However, mixing is a good solution for many families and children appear to have as much chance at becoming bilingual as those children brought up with an OPOL family. Mixing can follow on from more rigid or 'strict' strategies such as OPOL, once they are well established, or when the children prefer to mix rather than strictly separate each language.

Multilingual families are common around the world, especially in the Middle East, Asia and India, where several languages or dialects often overlap in one geographical area. Singapore is an example of a multilingual country. It has a mixed population of workers who emigrated from several countries, along with their languages. Officially English, Mandarin Chinese, Tamil and Malay are spoken, along with several other Chinese and Indian dialects. With mixed marriages and new immigrants arriving in the country, the linguistic mix can be varied. In *mixed multilingual* families, children especially need to know when to use each language because each language may be alternated, reserved for certain people, places or times or mixed all together in one phrase. The real challenge is for the children to work out which language to use appropriately and children generally pick up the linguistic 'rules' of their family quickly. There might be a clear separation of school/home languages or with certain people.

Mixed (bilingual)

A mix of two languages within the family

Both parents speak Language A & B fluently

The parents talk to their children in A or B (may alternate or mix languages)

Together the parents speak Language A or B (may alternate or mix languages)

The family lives in country using Language A or B, or both

Children attend school in Language A or B, or a bilingual school.

Children most likely to mix
Siblings most likely to mix

Positive:	Children learn to switch languages rapidly and have better vocabulary in both languages because they can talk about anything in either language.
Negative:	Mixing is not always appreciated by monolinguals (e.g. teachers and doctors) and young children must learn to not mix inappropriately, or not to be lazy by replacing difficult words with an easy one from the other language.

Mixed (multilingual)

A mix of three or more languages within the family
One parent speaks Language A, B and/or C to children One parent speaks Language A, B and/or C to children
Together the parents speak using Language A, B or C
The family lives in country using any of the three languages, A, B or C
Children most likely attend school in language of the country, A, B or C Siblings will most likely use language of the school and/or mix of other two within family.

Positive:	The children generally become multilingual, and are able to communicate with wide range of people.
Negative:	Children do not always learn to read or write in all three dialects or languages.

MINORITY-LANGUAGE-AT-HOME (ML@H)

One language at home, one language outside

The home-based strategy *minority-language-at-home* strategy (coded as *mL@H*) restricts language use in the home to one language, which is not a country language. When one parent chooses to speak his or her second language to support a parent this parent must be bilingual, at a high enough level that they can converse on all subjects with their children and understand family conversations (see Fantini and Caldas). The success of the strategy depends greatly on the language skills and cultural knowledge of the language they choose. There is usually a good reason why families choose such a strategy. Some parents chose it as preparation for the child's future education, or an option to move to another country at some time or to maintain a heritage language that might have been lost.

Minority-language-at-home

> One parent speaks Language B to children (their first language)
>
> Other parent speaks Language B to children (usually their second language)
>
> Together the parents speak Language B
> The family lives in country using Language A
>
> Children most likely attend school in La nguage A
> Siblings will most likely speak Language B while at home, Language A together
>   once they start school.
>
> Positive: Establishing early language B use.
>
> Negative: Once school and outside world become important to the child the
>   strategy is hard to maintain.

LINGUA FRANCA

Using a second or third language to communicate in

The *Lingua Franca* strategy, meaning 'the common language' or language of communication describes two parents who do not speak each other's language and use a third language together. The parents might follow an OPOL strategy and the children usually pick up the 'common' language of parental communication too.

Lingua franca: Two parental languages and one language between the parents

> One parent speaks Language A to children
>
> One parent speaks Language B to children
>
> Together the parents speak Language C,
>
> The family lives either a country using Language C or one of the parental languages
>
> Children most likely to attend school in language of country
> Siblings most likely to use school language together
>
> Positive: The children will hear three languages from early age and usually
>   become trilingual.
>
> Negative: The two parental languages need lots of support from extended family
>   or extra practice.

NON-NATIVE

Using a second language with your children

Like *minority-language-at-home*, this strategy demands that one or two parents choose to speak his or her second language with their children. The parent(s) must be bilingual, at a high enough level that they can converse on all subjects with their children and understand family conversations (see Saunders). The success of the strategies depends greatly on the language skills and cultural knowledge of the language they choose. There is usually a good reason why families choose such a strategy. Some parents chose it as preparation for the child's future education, or an option to move to another country at some time or to maintain a heritage language.

Non-native (one parent)

One parent speaks Language A to the children
One parent speaks Language B (his or her second language) to the children

Together the parents speak Language A or B
The family lives in country using Language A

Children most likely attend school in Language A
Siblings will most likely use Language A (some B)

Positive: Can give child a linguistic boost that he would not get through only schooling or classes.

Negative: Big commitment and one parent must stick at it long-term for results.

Non-native (both parents)

Both parents speak Language B to children (usually their second language)

Together the parents speak Language B
The family lives in country using Language A

Children most likely attend school in Language A
Siblings will most likely speak Language B while at home, Language A together once they start school.

Positive: As above, can give child a linguistic boost that he would not get through only schooling or classes.

Negative: Big commitment and both parents must stick at it long-term for results. May end up mixing languages sooner or later, or one parent might abandon if family communication is limited.

TIME AND PLACE

A regular time or location for language development

This strategy is linked to a place – a school, summer camp, after-school activity or visiting family in a country using another language. It can also be a time, like a school holiday, a summer break or even at the weekend. The parents are speaking one language together, while the other language is maintained by other people. The strategy can work if the child is motivated and there is enough time for practice. Can also be used to introduce or maintain a third or fourth language.

Time and Place

One parent speaks Language A
One parent speaks Language A

Together the parents speak Language A

The family lives in country using Language A

Children most likely attend school or organized activity in Language B
Siblings will most likely use Language A

Positive: Language is learnt in an informal fun setting and has clear boundaries. Ideal for learning a third or fourth language.

Negative: Depends on the child's motivation and time invested (often by parents) in the language learning environment to make it worthwhile.

	Strategy	Parents' language	Parent to children	Parent to parent	Country language	School activities	Child to child
1	OPOL (Majority)	A	A	A	A	A	A
		B	B				some B
	OPOL (Minority)	A	A	B	A	A	A/B
		B	B				
	OPOL (Mixed)	A	A	A & B	A	A	A
		B	B				some B
	OPOL + 1	A	A	A or B	C	C	A, B or C
		B	B				
2	Mixed	A & B	A & B	A & B	A or B	A or B	A & B
	Bilingual	A & B	A & B				
	Mixed	A, B or C	A, B or C	A, B or C	A, B or C	A, B or C	A, B or C
	Multilingual	A, B or C	A, B or C				
3	mL@H	A	B	A or B	A	A	B at home
		B	B				A outside
4	Lingua franca	A	A	C	A or B or C	A, B or C	A, B or C
5	Non-native (one)	A	A	A	A	A	A
		A	B				some B
	Non-native (both)	A	B	A	A	A	A/B
		A	B				
6	Time and Place	A	A	A	A	B	A

Appendix 2
The Online Survey

To find out what bilingual and multilingual families around the world thought about siblings I needed to collect data on their language use and their thoughts on being a bilingual family. I wanted a wide variety of international families with two or more children, following different strategies, with different age ranges of children and a mix of languages. How could I find such a sample group of families who represent real families? The answer was the internet. In the five years since I wrote my first book, in 2003, the internet has grown to become one of first points of reference for young families needing advice. Several sites have been created to help and inform bilingual, bicultural and multilingual families (for recommended sites see the Websites & Chat forums section in this book). The solution I chose was an online survey; so parents could complete the survey in their own time and there was no need for printing or posting. I set up my anonymous survey at SurveyMonkey.com, for three months. This was linked to my blog on Siblings & Bilingualism, which explained the survey. The link to the survey website was posted on the homepages of international bilingual and multilingual websites, in the quarterly newsletter *The Bilingual Family Newsletter*, and via friends and colleagues who passed on the link to other families they knew. In total 125 families responded and filled in the survey online. I had to exclude 20 families, either because they stopped mid-way through the survey, or they had two children too young to be judged on their language skills. In total I was able to use the data of 105 families. The online survey proved to be an effective way to reach a wide number of multilingual families around the world.

LOCATION AND NATIONALITY OF THE FAMILIES

Where were the families living? The families were from all around the globe, with the largest representations from families living in the United Kingdom and North America (Figure A.2.1). This was to be expected because the English-language parenting websites and publications were based in these countries. In Britain there were 35 families in total, mainly residing in the London area, or the southern part of England. In North America there were 20 families, from Chicago and Washington or from the states of California, Florida, North Carolina and Texas. Smaller numbers were recorded (three to ten replies) from families living in Germany, Singapore, Malaysia, France, Belgium and Wales. One or two families lived in Italy, Denmark, Spain, Netherlands, Czech Republic, Hungary, Norway, Sweden and Greece, Japan, Korea, Chile, Peru, Australia, Jordan, Israel and Ukraine.

How long had the parents lived in the current country of residence? I wanted to know if they were recent arrivals or established families living in their communities. This might mean that they might be more likely to choose a local school for education, as opposed to a private school in the other language or an international school (for more about the link between school language and bilingualism see Chapter 3). As the following chart shows (Figure A.2.2), a good percentage of families had been there for more than 10 years (40%), while a quarter (25%) had been there from five to ten years. There was a low count of short-term residents, both for those living there from one to three years (17%) or between three to five years (18%). The results on time of residence showed that most of the families in the survey were settled and would have strong ties to their local community.

Looking at the parent's nationality, there was a wide range of language couplings. From the 105 families who gave details about their nationality two-thirds of the families

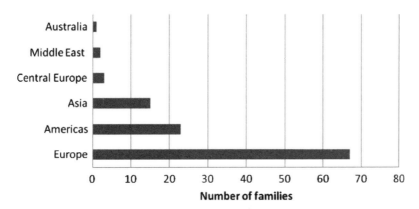

Figure A.2.1 Location of families

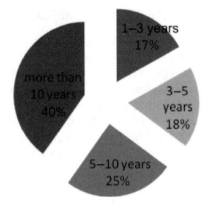

Figure A.2.2 Time spent in country of residence

had either an English-speaking British, American, Canadian or Australian parent (either the mother or the father).

Anglophone partner	65
Non-Anglophone couples	18
Same nationality couples	22

Of these 65 Anglo-mixed families, 22 had a French partner, 14 German and five Spanish partners. If the mother was English, American or Australian, she tended to live away from her country of origin. These mothers lived in Germany, France, Korea, Japan, Peru or Mexico. However, if the father was English or American he was most likely to be found in England or America (or another English-speaking country such as Singapore). There were also 18 families who did not have an English connection, with mixes like Dutch/Italian or French/Hungarian. Within this group nine parents had dual-nationality such as Swiss-French, Canadian-Lebanese, or Brazilian-Israeli. There were also 22 families where the parents both had the same nationality. Most of these families were expatriate families living abroad.

THE PARENTS AND THEIR LANGUAGE SKILLS

Who completed the survey? Around two-thirds of the parents were mothers in their thirties, and a quarter of the mothers were in their forties. In terms of education, nearly all (89%) of the respondents had been educated up to university level, while the other parents had completed studies up to school or college level. Twenty-eight parents worked in the field of Education, in private and public systems, either as English as a Second Language teachers, foreign language teachers, elementary school and high school teachers, university professors or college lecturers. There were 33 mothers who described themselves as stay-at-home moms, homemakers or house-wives. Many of these stay-at-home mothers were also working part-time from home, in translating, interpreting, part-time teaching or voluntary work. Another 39 parents worked in diverse areas such as PR, counseling, journalism, finance, computing, IT, software, law and office management. One hundred out of the 110 online responses were from mothers, because it was generally the mothers who visited the websites for bilingual families, or were involved in the online chat rooms. However, the views of both parents were encouraged and the parent completing the survey was asked to evaluate their partner's language skills and give joint opinions on their children's language use.

What languages did the parents speak? All in all, the parents spoke nearly 50 languages or dialects between them. In alphabetical order these were Afrikaans, Arabic, Bahasa Indonesia, Bahasa Malayu, Bangali, Burmese, Cantonese, Catalan, Creole, Croatian, Czech, Danish, Dutch, English, Finnish, French, German, Greek, Hainanese, Hebrew, Hindi, Hokkien, Hungarian, Ibo, Indonesian, Irish, Italian, Japanese, Korean, Malagasy, Mandarin, Mixteco, Nepali, Norwegian, Oriya, Portuguese, Punjabi, Romanian, Russian, Slovak, Spanish, Swedish, Tagalog, Teochew, Turkish, Urdu and Welsh.

All the mothers reported that they spoke at least two languages. The most common first (or strongest) language was English (32) followed by French (23) and German (13). There were smaller representations of Spanish (6), Portuguese (5), Italian (4) and Danish (3). The other languages were represented by one or two mothers. For three quarters of the mothers, English was their second language. German, French and Spanish were other second languages for mothers too, reflecting their partner's language or country of residence. Interestingly, 67% of the mothers spoke a third language and 37% had a fourth language. Third or fourth languages were typically French, Spanish and German, often linked to school or university studies. Otherwise, the third or fourth language tended to be a dialect or a language acquired as an expatriate.

For the fathers it was a similar story, with 89% of the fathers being able to speak a second language. The most common first (or strongest) language for half of the fathers was English (48), followed by French (9) and German (9). There were also some Spanish speakers (6), Dutch (4) and Italian, Portuguese (3) and Danish-speakers (3). Other languages were represented by one or two fathers. For the other fathers who were not Anglophone the most common second language was English. Like the mothers, French, Spanish, Italian and German were popular second, third and fourth languages. Half of the fathers could speak a third language too and 23% were quadrilingual.

We have to take these findings into context and remember that in many cases a parent might only have a basic or intermediate knowledge of one or more languages. I do not know if they use their languages regularly or whether they can communicate with a native speaker of that language. Many parents pick up a rudimentary understanding of a language from being the wife or husband of a local person, or living in a country for a few years. Some parents might have counted languages that they might have learnt previously at school, through work or through foreign language studies. I was not able to get more detailed information on the exact level of each parent's language skills in this brief survey. However, it is very positive that so many parents see themselves as bilingual or trilingual, and this is an excellent role model for their children.

I also asked which language(s) each parent spoke to their children and as a couple. The parents were asked to define their language strategy (OPOL, mL@H or a mixed strategy). This information on parent/child language use was essential for the chapter on language strategies and the parent's language use (for more on strategies see Chapter 2 and Appendix 1).

THE SIBLING SETS

How many children were involved in the survey? I collected data on 239 children, who were recorded in the survey, regarding their language skills, age, gender and number of children in each family. The age range of the children was very wide, going from 3 to 33 years of age. I did not give an upper-age limit because I wanted to hear from parents with older children and 10% (24) of the children were born in the 1970s or 1980s. These older children are now in their 20s or 30s, studying at university or living away from home. They would have a different perspective to the younger ones who are still under the care of their parents, although I still used some of their data in the survey. The graph below shows the year of birth for children born after 1990. Of the 95 first-born children numbers peaked in 2000, while the peak of the 85 second-born children was in 2005. There were only 18 third-born children, who were spread along the time frame, with between one and three births per year (Figure A.2.3).

I requested that parents did not give data for children younger than three years old, unless they could talk and be assessed on their verbal abilities. Nonetheless, several parents reported on their two-year-old children (those born in 2005 or 2006).

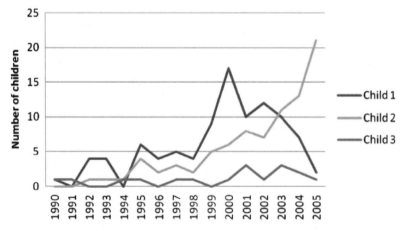

Figure A.2.3 Year of birth

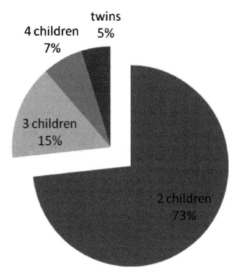

Figure A.2.4 Sibling sets

I excluded these young children from the online survey data, simply because it was difficult to judge if such a young child had sufficient language experience to make reliable and valued findings regarding their development. However, I have included selected parent's comments on their very young siblings in the book and in the *Family Profiles* section where the parents were interviewed by telephone or via email.

I grouped the children into sibling sets of two, three or four children (Figure A.2.4). The majority of families (73) had two children, which is quite typical of European and North American families. In a few cases there were two sets of siblings living in the same house, from two parents who had remarried and the children had step-sisters or brothers. There were five families with four children. This information was used for the discussion on age, family size and bilingualism (see Chapter 4). There were also five sets of twins (see Chapter 8 for more on twins).

What was the gender of the children? There were 121 boys and 118 girls, which were almost equally balanced, for the first, second and third children, with slightly less females in each group (Figure A.2.5). Curiously, nearly all of the fourth children were girls (see Chapter 5 for more on gender).

PARENT'S OPINIONS

What did the parents think about their children's language skills? Were the children able to speak two languages at the same level, or did they have one strong language and one weaker language? Could some children speak three languages? I asked the parents to rate up to four children's language use as Fluent, Intermediate or Beginner

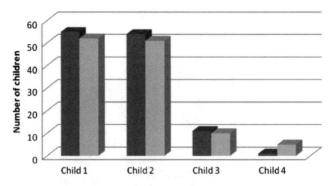

Figure A.2.5 Gender of children

(in a maximum of three languages). Understandably, this was only a very general guide to each child's individual language ability, which can change day-by-day depending on the situation they are in. Nevertheless, for the 225 children whose parents gave an assessment (not all the parents graded their children) we can have a 'snapshot' idea of how each child is communicating, according to their place in the family.

Sixty percent of the first-born children were equally fluent in two languages and could be described as balanced bilinguals. The other 40% of the firstborn children had an intermediate level in their second language, or a weaker second language, and could be described as emerging bilinguals. Beginner-level third language skills were common, since many children were learning a third language at school or through living in a foreign country. Overall, third language use was quite low, in line with the predominately younger age-span of the children. However, there were seven older grown-up or teenage children who were fluently trilingual.

For the second-born children, there was a slightly different story. Not all the children had gained complete fluency in their first-language yet. Around 80% of them had first-language fluency, while nine were described as intermediate or, in eleven cases, at a beginner level. This was probably because of their young age and limited verbal skills compared to an older sibling. We should bear in mind that in a few months or years it could be a different picture. The ratio of second-born children who were fluently bilingual was similar to the first-borns; around 50% of them could speak two languages well. Meanwhile, another 25% were on their way, and had an emerging or weaker second language. Around a quarter of the second children were at beginner level with their second language. This would be expected though, due to the young age of most of the second siblings. There was the same number of fully trilingual children as in the first-borns, and they were all older children. The third-borns were a much smaller group of just 20 children, of whom six were very young (aged four and under), and two were born after 1990. It was difficult to make judgments on their language skills, because so many of them were still developing their language skills. This information was used in relation to language order (see Chapter 4).

I also wanted to know what the parents thought about their children's language development and if they had changed their language use along the way. A series of multiple choice questions were posed for each child. Questions involved parents considering, with allowance for age, which of their children had the widest vocabulary, the most imagination, or the most 'correct' language use. These answers were used for data on birth order (see Chapter 6). I also asked the parents some open questions to find out if they had any children who mixed languages, refused to speak a language, had language-related problems or had a sibling who talked for another. Parents could reply in as much detail as they wished. These responses were used in the chapters on family size (see Chapter 4) and individual differences (see Chapter 7).

To end the survey the parents were requested to agree or disagree with four statements:

- Establishing bilingualism is easier when you only have one child.
- The first-born child is likely to be the most successful at becoming bilingual.
- An older child will usually help teach a younger child to speak a language.
- A girl will usually be more successful at becoming bilingual than a boy.

Glossary

Age gap: the difference in age between children in same family.

Bicultural: child or adult who engages equally with two cultures.

Bilingual: child or adult who speaks and understands two languages. They may well be able to read and write in both languages too, but this is not always the case.

Biliterate: child or adult who reads and writes in both languages.

Birth order: a child's place in the family – first, second, middle or last child.

Child-to-child language use: the language children choose when talking together in private.

Close-in-age siblings: siblings with three or less years between them.

Codeswitching: changing languages within the same sentence, either by inserting words from the other language or switching mid-sentence. It is grammatically correct in both languages and is often used between two or more bilinguals who understand both languages. Codeswitching can be influenced by the topic of conversation and shared experiences of the bilinguals.

Communicative anxiety: feeling nervous about speaking, often seen in introverted people.

Country language: the language of the country where the family lives, which often becomes the child's first or strongest language.

Dominant language: one language which is used more than the other one on a daily basis. It is often the school or country language.

Extrovert: a general description in language terms of a child or adult who is chatty, communicative and confident when talking.

Family language strategies: ways of organizing languages between family members (see also **one-parent–one-language, minority-language at home mixed, lingua franca, time and place).**

Foreign language anxiety: feeling nervous about speaking a foreign language.

Gender stability: the stage when the children understand the concept of gender and behave in gender-specific ways linked to the society they live in.

Immersion: intense period time spent using another language, either in a school, on holiday or with family and friends.

Introvert: a general description of a child or adult who is less inclined to chat or talk, especially in public.

L1: first language.

L2: second language.

L3: third language.

Language acquisition: refers to how children informally 'acquire' or learn a language from their parents and community in their early years.

Language bath: time spent in a country immersed in a language and culture, usually with close family or friends.

Language differentiation: the stage when a child understands that it has two languages available for communication and begins to separate them mentally and verbally.

Language friction: using language in a negative way to upset, taunt or insult each other.

Language gifted: a child who is able to use two or more languages fluently.

Language history: a chronological time line of when languages were acquired.

Language interaction: the linguistic communication between people.

Language order: listing of a child or adult's strongest or most fluent language, which is listed as first, second, third, etc.

Language patterns: the established ways of communication which suit the language needs of all family members. This can include mixing, language separation or a lingua franca. Second or later-born children often arrive in a home with a recognizable language pattern.

Language refusal: refusal or resistance to use a certain language. Often seen in young children and adolescents who will not use one language for various reasons.

Lingua franca: a common language, such as English, used for communication.

Lingua franca strategy: couples who speak different languages and use a third one for communication.

Majority-language: a language with a relatively higher prestige. Also used in this book to refer to the language used in the community where the family lives (see also **country language).**

Minority-language: a lower status language. Also used in this book to refer to the language spoken by the parent living outside their country (see also **parental language)**.

Minority-language-at-home: both parents choose to speak the minority-language together and to their children at home. Also known as **mL@H.**

Mixed strategy: parents who are bilingual mix both languages together on a daily basis. Mixing is linked to the situation and changes to suit the topic or group language needs.

Mixing: a term used by some authors to refer to young children who mix two languages, either by inserting words from the other language or switching languages mid-sentence. Children can use it as a way to communicate with other bilinguals, or they may use words that they do not yet know the equivalent for (see also **codeswitching**).

Monocultural: a child or adult who has one culture linked to their language.

Monolingual: a child or adult who is able to speak and understand one language. They can usually read and write in this language, but not always.

Motherese: The simplified version of speech that parents use when talking to a baby or young children.

Multilingual: a child or adult who speaks three or more languages.

Non-native strategy: one or both parents with the same language and culture who decide to bring up their children from birth using another language.

One-person–one-language/one-parent–one-language: Grammont's term for the method of bringing up children bilingually where each person or parent only speaks their language to the child, ensuring pure language input and a strong parent–child bond. Also known as **OPOL.**

OPOL–ML: strategy where the parents use the majority-language or country language between themselves.

OPOL–mL: strategy where the parents use the minority-language of one parent living away from their country between themselves.

OPOL + 1: strategy where the parents use two languages at home and live in a country where another language is used.

Parental language: a language used by a parent to a child.

Parental language strategies: the decision made by parents as to how they will bring up their children bilingually (see also **family language strategies**).

Passive bilingual: a child or adult who has knowledge of two languages but only uses one. This may be because one or two languages are not developed or lack practice or opportunity to use.

Sequential bilinguals: children learning a second language after one language is already established.

Siblings: the children in the family, which includes adopted, fostered, or step-brothers and sisters.

Sibling rivalry: the tensions and arguments between siblings.

Simultaneous bilinguals: children brought up with two languages from birth or from a very early age.

Strategies: see also **family language strategies**.

Time and place strategy: language learning and practice are linked to a certain place, such as a holiday home, or a time, like an extracurricular class.

Tricultural: a child or adult who identifies with three cultures.

Trilingual: a child or adult who speaks three languages.

Trilingual/multilingual strategy: parents who are using three or more languages with their children on a daily basis.

Wider age gap: siblings with three or more years age difference.

Websites and Chat Forums

Websites	Keywords
http://www.bilingualfamilynewsletter.com Quarterly paper newsletter for bilingual families. Archive online for subscribers.	Bilingual Family Newsletter
http://www.multilingual-matters.com Publisher of books and journals on bilingualism and multilingualism	Multilingual Matters
http://www.multilingualliving.com/index.html International advice on bilingualism	Multilingual Living
http://www.multilingualliving.com/magazine.html Online magazine available through bicultural family website	Multilingual Living Magazine
http://www.multilingualfamily.co.uk UK-based website with language specific links	Multilingual Family
http://www.geocities.com/bilingualfamilies/ Australian-based network for bilingual families	Bilingual Families Perth
http://www.nethelp.no/cindy/biling-fam.html Information on bilingualism	Bilingual Families Web Page
http://egung.myweb.uga.edu Information on bilingualism	Bilingual Parenting
http://humanities.byu.edu/bilingua/ Website for families using non-native strategy	Bilingual Parenting in a Foreign Language
http://www.twinslist.org/ Information on twins/multiples with section for multilingual families	Twinslist

Continued

Websites	Keywords
http://www.bilingualoptions.com.au/ Information on speech pathology (compiled by author Susanne Döpke)	Bilingual Options
http://www.ilovelanguages.com/index.php Links to wide number of languages and information on linguistics	I Love Languages
http://www.languagesonline.org.uk/ Site where children can practice language skills online	Languages Online
http://www.bilingualwiki.com Ongoing encyclopaedia on bilingualism	Bilingual Wikipedia
http://www.bilingualism-matters.org.uk University of Edinburgh site with information on bilingualism	Bilingualism Matters
http://www.cal.org/topics/ Information on bilingualism	Centre for Applied Linguistics (USA)
http://www.cafebilingue.com French-based international group called 'café bilingue' with forums and local groups	Café Bilingue/Enfants Bilingue
http://www.bilingualbabies.org Website and chat forum for parents with young children	Bilingual Babies
http://www.babycentre.co.uk UK-based website and chat forum for parents with babies. Group for multilingual families	Babycentre
http://www.bilingualfamiliesconnect.com International articles/forum	Bilingual Families Connect
http://www.multilingualchildren.org International articles/forum	Multilingual Children

Recommended Books for Bilingual Families

Baker, C. (2007) *A Parents' and Teachers' Guide to Bilingualism* (3rd edn). Clevedon: Multilingual Matters.

Barron-Hauwaert, S. (2004) *Language Strategies for Bilingual Families: The One Parent One Language Approach.* Clevedon: Multilingual Matters.

Caldas, S.J. (2006) *Raising Bilingual-Biliterate Children in Monolingual Cultures.* Clevedon: Multilingual Matters.

Cruz-Ferreira, M. (2006) *Three's a Crowd: Acquiring Portuguese in a Trilingual Environment.* Clevedon: Multilingual Matters.

Cunningham-Andersson, U. and Andersson, S. (1999/2004) *Growing Up with Two Languages: A Practical Guide.* London: Routledge.

De Houwer, A. (1990) *The Acquisition of Two Languages from Birth: A Case Study.* Cambridge: Cambridge University Press.

Deucher, M. and Quay, S. (2000) *Bilingual Acquisition: Theoretical Implications of a Case Study.* Oxford: Oxford University Press.

Fantini, A.E. (1985) *Language Acquisition of a Bilingual Child.* Clevedon: Multilingual Matters.

Grosjean, F. (1982) *Life with Two Languages: An Introduction to Bilingualism.* Cambridge, MA: Harvard University Press.

Harding, E. and Riley, P. (1986/2003) *The Bilingual Family – A Handbook for Parents.* Cambridge: Cambridge University Press.

Hoffmann, C. and Ystma, J. (eds) (2003) *Trilingualism in Family, School and Community.* Clevedon: Multilingual Matters.

Hua, Z. and Dodd, B. (2006) *Phonological Development and Disorders in Children: A Multilingual Perspective.* Clevedon: Multilingual Matters.

King, K. and Mackay, A. (2007) *The Bilingual Edge: Why, When and How to Teach your Child a Second Language.* New York: HarperCollins.

Lanza, E. (1997a) *Language Mixing in Infant Bilingualism: A Sociolinguistic Perspective.* Oxford: Oxford University Press.

Saunders, G. (1988) *Bilingual Children: From Birth to Teens.* Clevedon: Multilingual Matters.

Shin, S.J. (2005) *Developing in Two Languages: Korean Children in America.* Clevedon: Multilingual Matters.

Tokuhama-Espinosa, T. (2001) *Raising Multilingual Children: Foreign Language Acquisition and Children.* Westport, CT: Bergin & Garvey.

Wang, X. (2008) *Growing Up with Three Languages.* Clevedon: Multilingual Matters.

Yamamoto, M. (2001) *Language Use in Interlingual Families: A Japanese-English Sociolinguistic Study.* Clevedon: Multilingual Matters.

Zuer-Pearson, B. (2008) *Raising a Bilingual Child.* New York: Living Language/Random House.

References

Abu-Rabia, S. (2004) Teachers' role, learners' gender differences, and FL anxiety among seventh-grade students studying English as a FL. *Educational Psychology* 24 (5), 711–721.

Arnberg, L. (1987) *Raising Children Bilingually: The Pre-School Years*. Clevedon: Multilingual Matters.

Baker, C. (2007) *A Parents' and Teachers' Guide to Bilingualism* (3rd edn). Clevedon: Multilingual Matters.

Banerjee, R. (2005) Gender development. On WWW at http://www.open2.net/healtheducation/family_childdevelopment/2005/gender_development.html. Accessed 29.4.08.

Bank, S.P. and Kahn, M.D. (1997) *The Sibling Bond*. New York: Basic Books.

Barron-Hauwaert, S. (1999) Trilingualism – Issues surrounding trilingual families. Unpublished MEd dissertation, University of Sheffield, UK.

Barron-Hauwaert, S. (2000a) Trilingual families: Living with three languages. *The Bilingual Family Newsletter* 17 (1), 1–3.

Barron-Hauwaert, S. (2000b) Issues surrounding trilingual families – Children with simultaneous exposure to three languages. Paper presented at Innsbruck (Austria) Conference on Trilingualism and Third Language Acquisition. On WWW at http://zif.spz.tu-darmstadt.de/jg-05–1/beitrag/barron.htm. Accessed 29.5.09.

Barron-Hauwaert, S. (2002) The one-parent–one-language approach and its role in the bilingual family. Paper presented at Vigo (Spain) Symposium on Bilingualism.

Barron-Hauwaert, S. (2003) Trilingualism – A study of children growing up with three languages. In T. Tokuhama-Espinosa (ed.) *The Multilingual Mind*. Westport, CT: Praeger.

Barron-Hauwaert, S. (2004) *Language Strategies for Bilingual Families: The One Parent One Language Approach*. Clevedon: Multilingual Matters.

Barron-Hauwaert, S. (2007) Siblings and bilingualism. *Multilingual Living* – May/June 2007: 37–41.

Barron-Hauwaert, S. (2009) Siblings: A hidden influence in bilingual families. Paper presented at SOAS (London, UK) Conference: Multilingualism, Regional & Minority Languages: Paradigms for the Wider World.

Barton, M.E. and Tomasella, M. (1994) The rest of the family: The role of fathers and siblings in early language development. In C. Gallaway and B.J. Richards (eds) *Input and Interaction in Language Acquisition*. Cambridge: Cambridge University Press.

Biddulph, S. (1997) *Raising Boys*. London: Thorsons.

Benson-Cohen, C. (2005) Oral competence and OPOL: Factors affecting success. *The Bilingual Family Newsletter* 22 (4), 4–5

Bornstein, M.H., Leach, D.B. and Haynes, O.M. (2004) Vocabulary competence in first- and second-born siblings of the same chronological age. *Journal of Child Language* 31 (4), 855–873.

Bowen, C. (1999) Twins development and language. On WWW at from: http://www.speech-language-therapy.com/mbc.htm. Retrieved 24.11.08.

Brazelton, T.B. and Sparrow, J.D. (2005) *Understanding Sibling Rivalry: The Brazelton Way*. MA: De Capo Press.

Brewer, S. (2001) *A Child's World*. London: Headline Books.

Burman, D.D., Bitan, T. and Booth, J.R. (2008) Sex differences in neural processing of language among children. *Neuropsychologia* 46 (5), 1349–1362. See also: Northwestern University (2008) 'Boys' and girls' brains are different: Gender differences in language appear biological' *Science Daily*. On WWW at http://www.sciencedaily.com/releases/2008/03/080303120346.htm. Retrieved 13.10.08.

Caldas, S.J. (2006) *Raising Bilingual-Biliterate Children in Monolingual Cultures*. Clevedon: Multilingual Matters.

Chomsky, N. (1968) *Language and Mind*. New York: Harcourt Brace and World Inc.

Christensen, K., Petersen, I., Skytthe, A., Herskind, A-M., McGue, M. and Bingley, P. (2006) Comparison of academic performance of twins and singletons in adolescence: Follow-up study. *British Medical Journal* 333, 1095. On WWW at http://www.bmj.com/content/333/7578/1095.full. Accessed 25.11.06.

Cruz-Ferreira, M. (2006) *Three's a Crowd: Acquiring Portuguese in a Trilingual Environment*. Clevedon: Multilingual Matters.

Crystal, D. (1987) *The Cambridge Encyclopedia of Language*. Cambridge: Cambridge University Press.

Cunningham-Andersson, U. and Andersson, S. (1999/2004) *Growing Up with Two Languages: A Practical Guide*. London: Routledge.

Dale, P., Simonoff, E., Bishop, D., Eley, T., Oliver, B., Price, T., Purcell, S., Stevenson, J. and Plomin, R. (1998) Genetic influence on language delay in two-year-old children. *Nature Neuroscience* 1, 324–328.

Davies, B. (2004) The gender gap in modern languages: A comparison of attitude and performance in year 7 and year 10. *Language Learning Journal* 29 (1), 53–58.

De Houwer, A. (2005) Bilingual development in the early years. In K. Brown (ed.) *Encyclopedia of Language and Linguistics* (2nd edn). Oxford: Elsevier.

Dewaele, J.M. and Furnham, A. (2000) Personality and speech production: A pilot study of second language learners. *Personality and Individual Differences* 28, 355–365.

Dewaele, J.M., Petrides, K.V. and Furnham, A. (2008) The effects of trait emotional intelligence and sociobiographical variable on communicative anxiety and foreign language anxiety among adult multilinguals: A review and empirical investigation. *Language Learning* 58 (4), 911–960.

Döpke, S. (1992) *One Parent, One Language. An Interactional Approach*. Amsterdam: John Benjamins.

Dunn, J. and Kendrick, C. (1982) *Siblings: Love, Envy & Understanding*. MA: Harvard University Press.

Dunn, J. (1985) *Sisters and Brothers: The Developing Child*. MA: Harvard University Press.

Dunn, J. and Plomin, R. (1990) *Separate Lives: Why Siblings Are So Different*. New York: Basic Books.

Ernst, C. and Angst, J. (1983) *Birth Order: Its Influence on Personality*. Berlin: Springer-Verlag.

Eysenck, M.W. (1981) Learning, memory and personality. In H.J. Eysenck (ed.) *A Model for Personality*. Berlin: Springer-Verlag.

Faber, A. and Mazlish, E. (2004) *Siblings without Rivalry*. London: Piccadilly.

Fantini, A.E. (1985) *Language Acquisition of a Bilingual Child*. Clevedon: Multilingual Matters.

Garcia-Mendoza, V. (2008) What led us to these doors: Our family's journey of Bilingualism and International Adoption. *Multilingual Living* – July/August, 26–31.

Goodz, N.S. (1989) Parental language mixing in bilingual families. *Infant Mental Health Journal* 10, 25–44.

Grammont, M. (1902) *Observations sur le langage des enfants*. Paris: Mélanges Meillet.

Gregory, E. (1998) Siblings as mediators of literacy in linguistic minority communities. *Language and Education* 12 (1), 33–54.

Gregory, E., Long, S. and Volk, D. (2004) *Many Pathways to Literacy: Young Children Learning with Siblings: Grandparents, Peers and Communities*. London: Routledge.

Grover, M. (2005) The benefit of hindsight: The changing challenges of bilingual children. *The Bilingual Family Newsletter* 22 (4), 1–3.

Harding, E. and Riley, P. (1986/2003) *The Bilingual Family – A Handbook for Parents*. Cambridge: Cambridge University Press.

Harasty, J., Double, K.L., Halliday, G.M., Kril, J.J. and McRitchie, D.A. (1997) Language associated cortical regions are proportionally larger in the female brain. *Archives of Neurology* 54 (2), 171–176.

Harris, J.R. (1998) *The Nurture Assumption*. New York: W.W. Norton & Co.

Harris, J.R. (2006) *No Two Alike Human: Nature and Human Individuality*. New York: W.W. Norton & Co.

Helot, C. (1988) Bringing up children in English, French and Irish: Two case studies. *Language, Culture and Curriculum* 1 (3), 281–287.

Hoffmann, C. (1985) Language acquisition in two trilingual children. *The Journal of Multilingual and Multicultural Development* 6 (6), 479–495.

Horney, R. (2003) Bilingualism and adoption. 'Queries' section of *The Bilingual Family Newsletter* 20 (1), 6.

Horwitz, E.K. and Young, D.J. (1990) *Language Anxiety: From Theory and Research to Classroom Implications*. New Jersey, USA: Prentice-Hall.

http://www.census.gov/population/www/cen2000/briefs.html. Accessed 10.3.10.

http://www.usatoday.com/news/nation/2007-12-19-fertility_N.htm. Accessed 10.3.10.

http://europa.eu/rapid/pressReleasesAction.do?reference=MEMO/05/96&format=HTML&aged=0&language=EN&guiLanguage=en. Accessed 25.4.08.

http://www.pregnantpause.org/numbers/fertility.htm. Accessed 10.3.10.

Huss, L. (2003) Creating a bilingual family in a monolingual country. *The Bilingual Family Newsletter* 20 (3), 4–7.

Jisa, H. (2000) Language mixing in the weaker language. *The Journal of Pragmatics* 32 (1), 363–386.

King, K. and Mackay, A. (2007) *The Bilingual Edge: Why, When and How to Teach Your Child a Second Language*. New York: HarperCollins.

Kenner, C. (2004a) *Becoming Biliterate: Young Children Learning Different Writing Systems*. Stoke-on-Trent: Trentham Books.

Kenner, C. (2004b) Cantonese and Arabic-speaking pupils re-interpret their knowledge for primary school peers. In E. Gregory, D. Volk and S. Long (eds) *Many Pathways to Literacy*. London: Routledge.

Kohlberg, L. (1966) A cognitive-developmental analysis of children's sex role concepts and attitudes. In E. Maccoby (ed.) *The Development of Sex Differences*. London: Tavistock.

Kuebli, J., Butler, S. and Fivush, R. (1995) Mother–child talk about past emotions: Relations of maternal language and child gender over time. *Cognition and Emotion* 9 (2/3), 265–283.

Lanza, E. (1992) Can bilingual two-year-olds switch? *Journal of Child Language* 19, 633–658.

Laversuch, I.M. (2004a) International adoption and bilingualism. *The Bilingual Family Newsletter* 21 (3), 6–7.

Laversuch, I.M. (2004b) Speaking the language of the enemy. *The Bilingual Family Newsletter* 21 (4), 1–4.

Leaper, C., Anderson, K.J. and Sanders, P. (1998) Moderators of gender effects on parents' talk to their children: A meta-analysis. *Developmental Psychology* 34 (1), 3–27.

Leopold, W.F. (1939, 1947, 1949a, 1949b) *Speech Development of a Bilingual Child: A Linguists Record (in four parts)*. Evanston, IL: Northwestern Press.

Livingstone, T. (2005) *Child of Our Time*. London: Bantam Books.

Maccoby, E. (ed.) (1966) *The Development of Sex Differences*. London: Tavistock.

Majakari, N. (2006) In pursuit of my Finnish identity. *The Bilingual Family Newsletter* 23 (1), 6.

Martin, T. (2003) Multicultural adoption. *The Bilingual Family Newsletter* 20 (3), 2.

Nelson, K.E. and Bonvillian, J.D. (1978) Early language development: Conceptual growth and related processes between 2 and 4½ years of age. In K.E. Nelson (ed.) *Children's Language* (Vol. 1). New York: Gardner.

Obied, V. (2002) Sibling relationships in the development of biliteracy and emergence of a bicultural identity. Paper presented at *The Second University of Vigo International Symposium on Bilingualism*, Vigo, Spain, 2002.

Obied, V. (2009) How do siblings shape the language environment in bilingual families? *International Journal of Bilingual Education and Bilingualism* 12 (6), 705–720.

Pinker, S. (2002) *The Blank Slate*. New York: Allen Lane.

Plomin, R. (1990) *Nature and Nurture: An Introduction to Human Behavioral Genetics*. Pacific Grove, CA: Brooks/Cole.

Preuschoff, G. (2004) *Raising Girls*. London: Thorsens.

Ronjat, J. (1913) *Le développment du langage observé chez un enfant bilingue*. Paris: Champion.

Saunders, G. (1988) *Bilingual Children: From Birth to Teens*. Clevedon: Multilingual Matters.

Schuller, M. (2002) The language acquisition of twins and twin language. Paper from seminar Language Acquisition in its Developmental Context. On WWW at www.grin.com (Document No: V68267). Accessed 24.11.08.

Shin, S.J. (2002) Birth order and the language experience of bilingual children. *TESOL Quarterly* 36 (6), 103–113.

Shin, S.J. (2005) *Developing in Two Languages: Korean Children in America*. Clevedon: Multilingual Matters.

Slaby, R.G. and Frey, K.S. (1975) Development of gender consistency and selective attention to same-sex models. *Child Development* 46, 849–856.

Sulloway, J. F. (1997) *Born to Rebel: Birth Order, Family Dynamics and Creative Lives*. New York: Vintage Books.

Taeschner, T. (1983) *The Sun is Feminine: A Study on Language Acquisition in Childhood*. Berlin: Springer-Verlag.

The Times (UK) (2008) Older and wiser: Why· first-born children have higher IQ's. *The Times* 12 April, 4–5.

Time Magazine (2007) The secrets of birth order. *Time* 12 November, 32–38.

Tomasello, M. and Mannle, S. (1985) Pragmatics of sibling speech to one-year-olds. *Child Development* 56 (4), 911–917.

Tomosello, M., Mannle, S. and Kruger, A.C. (1986) Linguistic environment of 1- to 2-year-old twins. *Developmental Psychology* 22 (2), 169–178.

Tokuhama-Espinosa, T. (2001) *Raising Multilingual Children: Foreign Language Acquisition and Children*. Westport, CT: Bergin & Garvey.

Valenzuela, M. (2004) Family language strategies on the move: A balancing act. *The Bilingual Family Newsletter* 21 (4), 7.

Viding, E.M., Spinath, F.M., Price, T.S., Bishop, D.V.M., Philip, S., Dale, P. and Plomin, R. (2004) Genetic and environmental influence on language impairment in 4-year-old same-sex and opposite-sex twins. *Journal of Child Psychology and Psychiatry* 45 (2), 315–325.

Wang, X. (2009) Ensuring sustained trilingual development through motivation. *The Bilingual Family Newsletter* 26 (1), 1–6.

Warrington, M., Younger, M. and Williams, J. (2000) Student attitudes, image and the gender gap. *British Educational Research Journal* 26 (3), 393–407.

Williams, M., Burden, R. and Lanvers, U. (2002) French is the language of love and stuff: Student perceptions of issues related to motivation in learning a foreign language. *British Educational Research Journal* 28 (4), 503–528.

Wong Fillmore, L. (1991) When learning a second language means losing the first. *Early Childhood Research Quarterly* 6, 323–346.

Yamamoto, M. (2001) *Language Use in Interlingual Families: A Japanese-English Sociolinguistic Study.* Clevedon: Multilingual Matters.

Zajonc, R.B. (1976) Family configuration and intelligence. *Science* 192, 227–236.

Zuer-Pearson, B. (2008) *Raising a Bilingual Child.* New York: Living Language/Random House.

Index